Please return to
Paula Wurtz
480 759-4014

BOOKS BY FRANCINE PRINCE

•

The Dieter's Gourmet Cookbook

Diet for Life

Francine Prince's New Gourmet Recipes for Dieters

Francine Prince's Vitamin Diet for Quick and Easy Weight Loss

The Best of Francine Prince's Diet Gourmet Recipes

Francine Prince's Gourmet Recipes for Diabetics

Francine Prince's Quick and Easy Diet Gourmet Recipes

Feed Your Kids Bright

Francine Prince

Harold Prince, Ph.D.

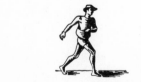

SIMON AND SCHUSTER

New York

This book is not intended, nor should it be regarded, as medical advice. For such advice, your doctor should be consulted.

For nutrition-related medical problems, a doctor trained and experienced in nutrition should be consulted.

Published by Simon and Schuster
A Division of Simon & Schuster, Inc.
Simon & Schuster Building
Rockefeller Center
1230 Avenue of the Americas
New York, New York 10020
SIMON AND SCHUSTER and colophon are registered trademarks of
Simon & Schuster, Inc.
Designed by Irving Perkins Associates
Manufactured in the United States of America

3   5   7   9   10   8   6   4

Library of Congress Cataloging-in-Publication Data
Prince, Francine.
Feed your kids bright.

Bibliography: p.
Includes index.
1. Children—Nutrition.   2. Intelligence—
Nutritional aspects.   3. Mood (Psychology)
4. Cookery.   I. Prince, Harold.   II. Title.
RJ206.P69   1986   649'.3   86-20373
ISBN 0-671-60522-4

Acknowledgment

To Fred Hills, our editor, for
his caring and brilliantly
creative guidance. We are most
grateful to him.

●

To
the bright kids
of today,
who will give us
the bright world
of tomorrow

Contents

9

Contents

Introduction

Four Revolutions to Brightness

Very quietly, without media hype or hoopla, over the last thirty years or so, four revolutions have occurred that could change the life of your kids and of every kid on earth.

They've happened in the school lunchrooms, in the clinics and laboratories of doctors, in the research facilities of a new breed of scientist—the neurobiologists, who study the biochemistry of the brain—and in the kitchen. They've occurred independently of each other, but taken together, they tell you, for the first time in history, how to bring up your kids healthy, happy, and bright with the help of the foods you feed them.

This is the story of those revolutions, and how you can use their breakthrough discoveries when you plan, shop for, and cook your family meals. Making the four revolutions—the work of thousands of the world's finest brains and of hundreds of thousands of work hours of innovative investigations—work for your kids is as simple as turning to page 134 right now. There you'll find the menus for the first days of eating bright.

The menus are practical—they're created almost entirely from supermarket foods. They're familiar—the dishes are mostly healthful taste-alike and look-alikes of American favorites. They're time- and labor-saving—each menu, with simple adaptations, serves the whole family, even when you're pregnant or breastfeeding. They're pleasurable transitions to a new way of eating that will feed you and your spouse right while they feed your kids to brightness.

What Is Brightness?

Brightness is not simply I.Q., although that's part of it; and the right diet has raised kids' I.Q.'s by as many as 35 points. Brightness is, among many subtle and splendid things, an awareness in the child of the emotional needs of others—an awareness that creates a child's affection, gentleness, helpfulness, and sense of humor. A bright child is a delight to be with.

Brightness is a friendly relationship with things, with the surrounding world and with the game of hide-and-seek it plays with kids: I'm hiding things from you, come and seek them out. Brightness is curiosity, the fascination with the unknown, the delight of probing, the joy of discovery—the discovery of a world in which the child lives without fear because the child knows it's understandable. Every bright child rediscovers the world so the child can live with it, friend-with-friend.

But friendly as the world is, it's filled with tricks and snares and puzzles—the everyday challenges of people and things that stand in the way of a child's untrammeled desires. It's the bright child who adjusts to the traps of reality that clamp down on desires, and knows deep down the limits of the possible. The bright child doesn't scream for the moon—or for a Twinkie. The bright child lives with the world as-is, content, serene—and makes the most of it.

Brightness is getting the most out of life; and getting the most out of life means selecting from all the wondrous things life has to offer, those things that please the child most. To find all the wondrous things life has to offer, the child must open door after door to new experiences—and that's learning. Learning is the key to making the most pleasurable selection from life's wonders—and the bright child knows this deep down. A bright child has no problems about learning. He—she—wants to learn more, faster, and more and more.

A bright child is at peace and peaceful. There is no urge to win at all costs, to beat out the other kids, to see life as conflict, to play king of the hill for real. But if success does come by effort and industry and service to others, the bright child accepts it gracefully without boasting or arrogance, and with the joy that comes with accomplishment. The bright child is a balanced child. A balanced child is a loving child. And a lovable one.

In harmony with people and things; confident in a world the child never made but has learned to understand, adapt to, and make the most of through learning; giving and receiving love, the bright child is a happy child.

Can the right diet evoke this remarkable child? Of course not. Genes are immutable. Parental influence is ponderous. Schools can be a passage to the stars, but they can also be straitjackets. Peer pressure is a mind-altering drug. Poverty is a foe of brightness. So is affluence. TV deprives the child of the mental stimulation without which brightness cannot mature. Some social climates, moral attitudes, standards of success can stifle brightness. The road to brightness is not a smooth one. But putting your child on that road with sound nutrition can help your child get over the rough spots. Help mightily.

The nutrition/brightness revolution in the schools has demonstrated that. With a switch of diet, Johnny *can* read, Jane *can* learn. The nutrition/brightness revolution in medical research has helped turn unhappy, miserable, unfit kids into happy-at-home and at-school winners via diet. Diet is responsible for the successful birth of the child's brain in the embryo, and of the astounding second birth of the brain in the newborn to ages 3 through 5, the neurobiologists who created the nutrition/brightness revolution in brain research report. And the same diet that makes kids healthy, the women of the nutrition/brightness revolution in the kitchen have discovered, can make kids bright.

In these pages you'll meet the heroes of these revolutions, including:

Sara Sloan, the educator/nutritionist, who first transformed kids from dull to bright on a mass scale by banning junk foods and replacing them with bright foods in the meal programs of two entire school systems.

Dr. Ben Feingold, who first successfully treated hyperactive kids by a diet free of certain foods that he found could adversely affect kids' brains.

Dr. Glen Green, who first discovered how a vitamin supplement could reverse early symptoms of a brain disorder; and Dr. Carl C. Pfeiffer, who was one of the first to achieve the same kind of result with a mineral supplement.

Dr. Allan Cott, who first created successful treatments for learning disabilities based on sugar-free, vitamin/mineral-supplemented diets.

Dr. William G. Crook, who first turned slow learners around by the elimination of a group of brain-harmful foods that he discovered.

Dr. Jean-Pierre Changeux, the eminent neurobiologist who first created the basic scenario for brain growth, providing the scientific basis for the new nutritional approaches to feeding kids bright from preconception to adolescence.

Dr. Ralph Minear, who first developed a practical nutritional program for the best possible growth and performance of a child's brain.

And the pioneers who created the nutrition/brightness revolution in the kitchen—the eminent nutritionists, Alice White and Dorcas Demasio; and one of the authors of this book, Francine Prince— who translated the science of the nutrition/brightness revolutions into bright meals for kids and right meals for their parents.

You'll learn from the breakthroughs of all these innovators, and from the achievements of men and women like them, the *why* of feeding your kids bright. Hard-core science, not talk-show science, this is the stuff of symposia and scientific journals, of formulas and tables and charts, of laboratory analyses and computer input/output; but it's presented here in a language as simple as your morning newspaper's. Knowing the *why* of the care of your kids is your inalienable right as a parent. There is no other way you, in collaboration with your child's doctor, can come to a reasonable decision about the physical and mental welfare of your child.

You'll learn *how* the nutrition/brightness revolutions bettered the lives of vast numbers of children throughout the world, and of individual kids in the United States—kids who could be very much like yours. You'll meet kids with names and faces and individual personalities, who might have been sedated and institutionalized were it not for the simple nutritional ways that terminated their brain dysfunctions. You'll witness the way kids, suffering from the plethora of learning disabilities from hyperactivity to symptoms of schizophrenia, have been restored to mental health, and then advanced to brightness, through nutrition.

Most importantly, you'll learn how you can help protect your child—starting even before conception—from the tragic epidemic of children's mental disorders that is sweeping the nation, and bring up your child bright instead. The *how* is an eating plan, presented for the first time in this book, based on these sound principles that have emerged from the nutrition/brightness revolutions:

- Your child's brain is a biochemical machine. It's built on biochemicals. It grows on biochemicals. It works on biochemicals.

- There's only one way your child can get those biochemicals—from the right nutrients in the right amounts.

- There's only one way your child can get the right nutrients in the right amounts—from a new kind of diet; for you, from preconception through pregnancy and breastfeeding, and for your child, from infancy to adolescence.

- It's a diet that generates the full quota of biochemicals your child's brain needs to develop to its peak potential for thinking, for feeling, for acting—for brightness.

The diet is our Eating Plan for Brighter Kids—the cornerstone of which is the Basic All-Family Menu Plan—that's as healthful to your child's body as it is to your child's brain. Built on the foundations of the Federal Dietary Guidelines and the recommendations of the American Academy of Pediatrics for the nutritional care of mother and child, it incorporates all the major findings of the four nutritional revolutions accepted by mainstream nutrition physicians.

It's a diet that's easy to get used to because it includes familiar favorites—like whamburgers, frosty shakes, and french fries—only healthful ones. It's a diet for the whole family that's easily adapted to pregnancy and breastfeeding and the changing nutrition needs of your growing kids. It's a diet that goes on from familiar favorites to exciting new taste adventures. It's a delicious, healthful diet that you can cook—the menu plans and the recipes are all here—for feeding you and your husband right while feeding your kids bright.

The four nutrition/brightness revolutions come together in your kitchen. In your kitchen, you can revolutionize the lives of your kids.

PART

I

·———·

The Nutrition/ Brightness Revolution in the Schools

• CHAPTER •

1

"EAT TO LEARN! LEARN TO EAT!"

For School Kids: Food for the Body to Expand the Mind

If your kids have learning problems, will better food solve them?

Will eating breakfasts make your school kids brighter?

Will eating snacks?

Can junk foods be responsible for your kids' difficulties at school?

Can the right kind of lunch improve school performance?

How can *you* get your school kids to eat bright?

Sara Sloan, mainly as the director of Food and Nutrition Programs, fed 109 million kids over thirty-one years in the school systems of Columbia, South Carolina, and Fulton County, Georgia, and found the answers.

She switched her kids from the wrong foods to the right foods, from the wrong eating habits to the right eating habits—and the results were astounding:

Now Johnny could read. Johnny could sit still. Johnny could remember. Johnny could concentrate. Johnny could write. Johnny could complete assignments. Johnny could be quiet when quiet was called for. Johnny could build his vocabulary. Johnny could express himself. Johnny could stay with a subject for a long time. Johnny could *learn*. And so could Jane.

"Children were happier," says Sara Sloan. These were the kids who had been grouchy and irritable. Kids who had been depressed. Kids who had been hostile, aggressive. Kids who had acted goofy. Kids who had been nervous and moody. Kids who had flared up for no reason at all. Kids who had been pint-sized Jekyll and Hydes. "These were the kids who had made the classroom a combat zone," Sara Sloan says. "But now they were a delight to be with."

Fed right, the kids were healthier, too. Headaches, stomach up-sets, colds, allergies, vague teacher-I-don't-feel-good aches and pains sharply declined. So did visits to The Nurse. Tiredness, that blatant barometer of poor health (some kids were so chronically fatigued they couldn't even play), gave way to the normal high energy of childhood. Athletic instructors and coaches remarked on the upsurge of stamina and vigor. Kids who previously couldn't get through a lesson without drooping, were as fresh at the end of a school day as when it began.

Brighter, happier, healthier, Sara Sloan's kids were better equipped for childhood's greatest adventure: the exploration of the world around them in the school and outside of it. "The right foods," Sara Sloan says, "helped open the doors to interest, curi-osity, enthusiasm, imagination, motivation and the courage to try something new. The right teachers led them through the doors."

Here's how Sara Sloan created a revolution in school kids' eating patterns for breakfast, snacks, and lunch—how these patterns can help you help your kids to brightness—and how they form one of the solid foundations on which we've built our Eating Plan for Brighter Kids.

Bright Kids Eat Breakfast

In the school system of Fulton County, Georgia (Atlanta is the hub), there was an epidemic of "morning dopiness." There was no med-ical name for the disorder, the school doctors had no treatment for it, but the symptoms were putting stress on the teachers and dis-turbing the other kids. Dullness went along with restlessness, lack of interest with hostility.

Why only in the morning?

Sara Sloan found that many of the kids were not eating breakfast, and to her that was the explanation.

"A kid whose last meal is dinner the night before," she explains, "is going about sixteen hours without food, and that kid is *hungry*. Put a hungry kid in the classroom, and all the kid's going to be interested in is when am I going to eat, not reading, writing, and arithmetic. An empty stomach means an empty mind."

To prove her point, she introduced a nutritious morning snack into the classroom (there were no facilities for a full breakfast). Her Peanut Butter Balls are a well-balanced mini-meal. She taught teachers how to make them and the teachers taught the kids.

"As soon as the kids arrived at school," she says, "they mixed peanut butter with nonfat dry milk, shaped the mix into balls, and rolled them into crushed seeds. The kids had fun making them. The kids loved them."

Morning dopiness disappeared in many of the kids, and C's and D's began to turn into B's and A's. "Bright kids," says Sara Sloan, "eat breakfasts."

Sara Sloan came to that conclusion in 1965 when only one scientific test had been made on the effect of skipped breakfasts on children. But, although the test, conducted by the University of Iowa, and known as the Iowa Breakfast Studies, had reached conclusions similar to Sara Sloan's, it had limited the study to children of 12 years of age and older. Sara Sloan had established the no-breakfast/poor-performance link among school kids from kindergarten to junior high school—from ages 5 to 13.

Not until 1985 would *that* link be confirmed during a two-day symposium on "Diet and Behavior: A Multidisciplinary Evaluation," sponsored by the American Medical Association, the International Life Sciences Institute, and the Nutrition Foundation. The symposium concluded, as reported by the *Tufts University Diet and Nutrition Letter:*

"Breakfast-skipping on the part of youngsters appears to affect how well they perform in school. Recent research reinforces the importance of breakfast for children. Children made more mistakes on a test, or performed certain tasks more poorly, when breakfast was skipped."

Bright Kids Eat *Nutritious* Breakfasts

Many kids who ate breakfasts—"hearty breakfasts," their mothers said—also suffered from morning dopiness.

"But you know what kind of breakfasts they were eating?" Sara Sloan asks. "Kids' breakfast cereals. Junk-food breakfasts. Almost all sugar, almost no nutrition. Those kids were almost as nutrition-starved as the kids who ate no breakfast, and they behaved the same way. Junk-food breakfasts are as bad as no breakfasts at all."

Sara Sloan's Peanut Butter Balls helped these kids as well. But, useful as an expedient, they're no substitutes over the long run for real, nutritious breakfasts. That's the kind that's mandatory on our Eating Plan for Brighter Kids (and for parents, too, who also suffer from morning dopiness).

Because we know that preparing nutritious breakfasts can be a stress event in the A.M. hurly-burly when everyone has an eye on the clock, we've made our breakfast menus quick and easy. *And* more attractive for kids (and the rest of the family) than Peanut Butter Balls.

Bright Kids Eat Nutritious Snacks

In the early 1970s, a controversy was raging among health professionals about whether or not snacks were good for kids, with fashionable opinion leaning to they were not. But Sara Sloan had seen her morning Peanut Butter Balls work wonders for her kids, and she was on the side of snacks—the right kind of snacks.

"Kids really don't need snacks in the morning if they have a nutritious breakfast, but they do need them after school. That's the way kids are made," she says. "They get ravenous after school. There's nothing wrong with afternoon snacks. What was wrong was that kids were eating the wrong kinds of snacks."

Most snacks were junk foods. Not only the vending machines' irresistible array of sweets for kids but also Mom's commercial jam on processed white bread with chocolate milk. Sara Sloan was among the first to realize how badly junk-food snacks affect school performance—even though they're eaten after school.

"Sugar is in everything," she says, "and it's just terrible for kids. It gives them a lift after school—a burst of energy when they need it—but then it lets them down, depresses them. They get 'sugar blues'—and that's no state to be in when you have homework to do. And the sugar kills their appetite for dinner, and they miss all that nutrition."

Nutritious snacks must replace junk-food snacks, Sara Sloan decided. But astonishing as it is to health-oriented Americans of the late 1980s, in the early seventies there was not a single cookbook on junk-free snacks for kids, no set of guidelines, not even a list of suggestions. It wouldn't be until 1979 that the U.S. Department of Agriculture, as part of its observance of the International Year of the Child, would put its stamp of approval on groups of foods for kids from which sugar-free, junk-free snacks could be selected or made.

Sara Sloan was the pioneer creator of nutritious snacks for kids. From today's viewpoint, most seem unsaleable to kids (baked potato skins with marinated sprouts?), and some are actually not as nutritious as she thought (she recommends commercial whole-wheat crackers, for instance, apparently unaware of their heavy content of additives). But the step she took was in the right direction, and it was a giant step. All creators of nutritious snacks for kids have been inspired by her, as we have.

Her goal was snacks of high-energy, nutrient-rich ingredients that provide kids with the midafternoon lift they need—the natural lift that never lets them down, the kind that comes with good nutrition. That's the type of snacks we've built into our Eating Plan for Brighter Kids. But, unlike most nutritious snacks, they're easily saleable to kids; some actually look like and taste like the junk-food snacks today's kids have grown to love.

Bright Kids Don't Eat Junk Foods for Lunch

In 1951, when Sara Sloan started her career as a school nutritionist, there were few problem kids, she says. "We had some backward kids and some disturbed kids, but they were the exceptions. And I think this was true of most school systems of that time."

Aware of contrasting current statistics that characterize one out of five school kids as having some type of learning disability, she sees the distressing shift in children's eating patterns since the 1950s as a root cause. "It's hard to believe," she says, "that it's only in the last thirty-five years or so that processed foods have largely replaced natural foods."

She recalls that up to the early 1950s, natural foods were the American way of eating, and that's the way she fed her kids in the school lunchrooms. "We had a nutritional paradise," she says, "but in the rush and push to meet financial requirements, we lost it."

Natural-food lunchrooms became fast-food school cafeterias. "When I joined the school system," she says, "no one even dreamed that they would ever see junk food in a school lunchroom —but here it was. Burgers, fries, shakes. Foods with preservatives, additives, artificial colors and flavors. Lots of sugar and salt. Even salads were premixed. Chemicals were supposed to keep them fresh. But they didn't."

The effects on the kids were heartbreaking, she says. "We had vandalism. We had rowdiness in the lunchrooms. We had disciplinary problems, usually after lunch. We never, never, had those things happen before. Grades fell. So did reading scores. There were many cases now of kids who couldn't stop talking, and kids who threw temper tantrums. There were too many depressed kids and kids suffering from chronic fatigue. More kids were visiting the nurse. There were more absentees because of sickness. Teachers said kids just didn't seem to be as healthy as they had been."

Sara Sloan's observations have been corroborated by a 1983 study conducted by Dr. Michael Colgan, a leading nutrition scientist and a visiting scholar at the Rockefeller University, New York. Coincident with the junk-food invasion, which began in the early 1950s and occupied most school lunchrooms by 1960, he wrote, "there had been a huge rise in the number of children with brain damage, hyperactivity, or learning disability. A study at the University of California suggests that the problem has doubled since the 1960s."

Enraged by the junk food–caused mental and physical deterioration of her school kids—"Nutritional abuse of kids is a form of child abuse," Sara Sloan says—she banned all junk food in the vending machines of the Fulton County school system. She started to de-junk lunchroom menus by prohibiting chocolate milk. "The sugar and caffeine just about wrecks kids in the afternoon."

Next, she eliminated typical schoolroom lunches like:

HAMBURGER ON WHITE ROLL
FRENCH FRIES
KETCHUP AND PICKLE SLICES
BROWNIE, AND
CHOCOLATE MILK

Every one of these items contains junk-food ingredients, she points out. The white bun and the brownie are made up almost entirely of bleached white flour and sugar. The hamburger and french fries contain too much animal fat. There are multiple additives in all foods. Salt is outrageously high in the pickles, and there is too much salt in everything, including the brownies and the chocolate milk. The ketchup is loaded with sugar.

"What is true of the hamburger lunch," Sara Sloan says, "is also true of most other standard school lunches. Anyone who takes the time to check charts of the nutrient contents of foods will find some ingredients harmful to kids in almost all the foods most schools serve."

She was the first to ban junk foods in the schools, a practice now followed by many school systems. "We don't permit pornographic books in the school libraries," she says, "why should we permit pornographic food in school lunchrooms?"

Sara Sloan replaced junk-food lunches with what she calls "Nutra Lunches," "Nutra" standing for Nutrition Naturally. This is a typical Nutra Lunch, which these days could very well be on the menu of a fashionable health-food restaurant:

SESAME CHICKEN
(SAUTÉED CHICKEN BREASTS SPRINKLED WITH SESAME SEEDS)
WHEAT GERM GRAVY
TOSSED SALAD WITH COTTAGE CHEESE DRESSING
CRACKED WHEAT BREAD
FRESH FRUIT
MILK

How You Can Get Your Kids to Switch to Healthful Foods

"You can lead kids to the table," mothers told Sara Sloan, "but you can't make them eat." So Sara Sloan devised several methods that worked for her multimillions of kids, and could work for your kids, too.

The simplest one, and one of the best for getting kids to try something new, was putting up this sign over the healthful dishes on the lunchroom counter: FOR ADULTS ONLY. "You couldn't keep the kids away from them," she says. It's a cute idea for starters, but over the long haul it's likely to wear thin, particularly if the kids don't like what they taste. Her other ideas have a more lasting impact.

Discovering that kids will eat anything they make themselves, she taught them how to cook. "What they cooked for themselves, no matter how awful it turned out the first time, and how messy they got themselves and everything else—they loved it," she says. "Cooking comes naturally to children of both sexes, if you just give them a chance and encourage them."

We think this is a great idea; every kid should learn how to cook —the bright way. That's why some of the recipes in this book are so easy that your kids can make them under your supervision. There's a list on page 261.

Let your kids learn by watching you cook and helping you cook. You'll be surprised how eager they'll be to imitate, then innovate. In one of Sara Sloan's schools, Miss Hinton's ardent kindergarten watchers-and-helpers came up with the idea of "smushing" cooked apples through a sieve and adding spices to make their own kind of applesauce.

Sara Sloan, who has collected a volume of her kids' culinary creations, is particularly fond of second-grader John Taylor's "Rocket Salad." The launching pad is a slice of pineapple on a bed of a crisp lettuce leaf; the rocket is half a peeled banana set upright in the center of the pineapple slice; and the nose cone is half a fresh cherry fastened to the top of the banana with a toothpick.

Sara Sloan also recommends that kids grow some of their own food. "Kids love to see things grow," she says, "particularly if they make them grow." She suggests vegetable gardens if you're in the suburbs or the country; or, if you're in a city apartment, sprouts grown in a jar. Sprouts are pretty messy to grow, but they grow fast, and they hold the younger kids' interest. "Kids who would never look at a vegetable or a sprout," Sara Sloan says, "eat them with as much relish as if they were Big Macs—when they grow them themselves."

She also advocates teaching kids about sound nutrition, the earlier the better. Cooking is one way, when you tell your kids *why* the foods you're making—or making together—are good for them. Don't be shy about spelling it out in terms of their own interests: "You'll have more fun. You'll make more friends. You won't get sick. You'll do better in school."

Take them shopping. Show them what's good and what's bad by

what you buy and what you don't. Even if your kids can't read yet, show them where the ingredients are listed on the package; and if the list is long, tell them the product is likely to be bad for them. If your kids can read, tell them that the strange words on the ingredients list mean "Don't Eat Me."

When your kids ask the inevitable "Why?" instruct them about the fundamentals of nutrition simply and clearly. If you can't do that now, you will when you finish this book; and that's one of the pressing reasons this book was written. *You* will have to instruct them, because most schools don't teach nutrition in the early grades.

"When I came to Fulton County, I remember asking a fourth-grade class, 'What are the four Food Groups?' " Sara Sloan says. "The kids answered, 'Pizza Hut. Burger King. McDonald's. And Arby's.' "

She advises you to put up a sign in your school kids' rooms, or on your refrigerator door, that says EAT TO LEARN! LEARN TO EAT!

"But in the final analysis it's the example you set that will put your kids on the right eating track or the wrong one," she warns. "If you feed your kids fruit for dessert while you and your husband gorge on ice cream, your kids will want ice cream, too. You have to set an example. You have to be a role model. Good nutrition is more caught than taught."

That's another reason our Eating Plan for Brighter Kids is an eating plan for the whole family, as delicious for you as it is for your kids, making your new role as your kids' teacher on eating for health and brightness easy to play.

A Junk Food–Free Diet Means Brighter Kids

There are no junk foods on Sara Sloan's Nutra Diet, only nonprocessed natural foods. The diet works well—so well that seventh-graders in her Fulton County school system at one time routinely dramatized its success with this mini-experiment:

White rats were the subjects because, as one student explained, "Rats react to foods much the same as humans but in a much shorter time." There were six animals in the experiment, and each was given a pet name. At the start, all were as bright and healthy as well-cared-for laboratory rats usually are.

Then:

Elmer and Lulu were fed only the kinds of snacks most American kids ate: candy, desserts, potato chips, and soft drinks. They became dopey, nervous, and irritable.

Dan's and Little Ann's menus were composed exclusively of hamburgers, fries, and soft drinks—the kind of food most kids were served at lunch in school cafeterias nationwide. This pair became fat, apathetic, and lost their mental alertness.

All four of those rats also fell ill. Their coats degenerated into raggedness, and their tails disrupted into scales and unsightly discolorations.

On the other hand, Rufus and Priscilla were fed nothing but Nutra food. They remained as clever and happy and full of vigor as they had been when the experiment began. Maybe a little more so.

The experiment ended happily for all the rats. When the rats on the junk-food diets were switched to the Nutra Program, they recovered completely, and the kids couldn't tell them apart from Rufus and Priscilla.

Endorsement of Sara Sloan's Nutra Diet has come from the three most prestigious decision-making groups in the nation concerned with children's health and education:

The United States Department of Agriculture (USDA), which has set up an "Anti-Junk-Food Policy," requiring school cafeterias to cease and desist from serving candy, potato chips, and soft drinks. The national Parent-Teachers Association (PTA), which has taken a stand against nonnutritive food in schools. And the International Reading Associations (IRA), representing 64,000 teachers throughout the globe, which is now urging parents to eliminate "foods that block learning" and replace them with "foods that are the building blocks of learning."

Many school systems throughout the country have adapted the Nutra Diet, with successes much like Sara Sloan achieved in her school systems. Kids switched off junk food were healthier and happier. They had greater attention span, could take directions without hostility, were better behaved in classrooms and lunchroom. Their reading scores went up, and so did their grades. They were brighter.

"I started a revolution," Sara Sloan says. "What I did was to awaken parents and teachers, and the kids themselves, to the danger of junk foods not only to kids' bodies but to kids' minds, and point the way to healthier, happier, and brighter kids with breakfasts, snacks, and lunches that contain no junk foods."

The slogan of Sara Sloan's revolution was "Food for the body to expand the mind."

The junk foods that did not meet that criterion, those that Sara Sloan banned, we have excluded from our menus. We have also updated her list of "forbidden" foods. Of the foods that were her favorites, we've retained those that meet today's more exacting standards set by the other nutrition/brightness revolutions.

Sara Sloan is the recipient of the prestigious Rachel Carson Award; and rightly so, for Sara Sloan is the Rachel Carson of children's nutrition. We have adapted the best of Sara Sloan's contributions as part of our Eating Plan for Brighter Kids.

The Nutrition/ Brightness Revolution in Medical Research

CHAPTER

2

SALICYLATES AND ADDITIVES

Foods That Could Make Your Kids Hyperactive

In the 1950s a strange new malady, now claiming some 5 million victims, began to rampage among American kids—hyperactivity.

The hyperactive child can't be still, not for more than seconds. With an attention span shorter than it takes to read a line of type, he can't learn. He goes on unstoppable verbal marathons. Irritated by almost anything, he responds with uncontrolled aggression. He's a malign Dennis the Menace. No classroom can withstand his violent disruptiveness. For reasons no one as yet can fathom, there are more "he's" among hyperactives than "she's."

Jonathan is a textbook hyperactive. His first-grade schoolteacher, a fifteen-year veteran, testifying in a suit to vacate a court order reversing her decision to expel Jonathan, said the 7-year-old "motor mouth" was beyond her control.

Jonathan seemed to be a brilliant child when the semester began. "He was very quick and had beautiful handwriting. I liked him very much. He used to come to my desk and talk. But by the second day," she told the court, "I noticed his mouth wouldn't stop moving." He talked all the time, even when he was disciplined by being made to stand alone in the corridor, or when he was sent to the Principal's office.

Uncontrollable as well was his impertinence and his disrespect. But what concerned his teacher most was his outbursts of violence. "He beats up other kids, including fifth-grade boys twice his size. I saw them doubling over in pain. He would hit, poke, kick, and bother the other children. He couldn't walk down the hall without shoving some other kid in front of him."

His effect on the class of sixteen was devastating. "The quiet ones became sullen. The gifted ones stopped working. The ones with the least control, lost it. . . . My class became a zoo."

Unable to restrain Jonathan or stay the court order reinstating him to her class, the teacher reached a point where, she said, she could no longer teach. "So I quit because of this one student."

Not every hyperactive is a Jonathan, a one-kid reign of terror. But even the mildest form of hyperactivity can be heartbreaking to parents and teachers, and life-shattering to a child. Your child is probably hyperactive if you find yourself checking off every symptom listed on the chart "Is Your Child Hyperactive?" (opposite).

But even if the answer is "no," your child could become hyperactive when certain amounts of foods that are in the diet of virtually every kid in America are consumed. Dr. Ben F. Feingold, the California pediatrician who made this path-breaking discovery, classifies the hyperactivity-inducing foods into two types: foods containing salicylates, and foods containing additives.

Protecting Your Kids from Salicylates

Dr. Feingold's discovery linking salicylate-containing foods to hyperactivity was, like so many other great scientific discoveries, serendipitous. He had observed that some hyperactive kids on aspirin were no longer hyperactive when taken off the drug. Aspirin is a member of a class of chemicals called salicylates.

But some kids who had never taken aspirin in their lives were also hyperactive. How to explain? With a brilliant flash of insight, Dr. Feingold searched for salicylates that occurred naturally *in foods.* He found them. When he removed the salicylate-containing foods from some hyperactives' diets, the disorder disappeared.

Dr. Feingold's therapy was adapted by hundreds of doctors with similar success. Dr. Allan Cott, perhaps the nation's foremost medical authority on hyperactivity, reported that he had "treated thousands of . . . kids [and] when the offending [salicylate-containing] foods were removed from the diet . . . the overwhelming majority improved quickly and significantly."

There's a list of salicylate-containing foods on page 38. If, after eating any of them, your kids become hyperactive, you can follow

Is Your Child Hyperactive?
• ——————————— •

A check in each box indicates the classic syndrome of hyperactivity. Any child may become hyperactive after consumption of trigger amounts of foods containing salicylates or additives.

☐ Can't sit still
☐ Can't keep quiet
☐ Learning difficulties
☐ Intensely aggressive
☐ Impertinent
☐ Disrespectful

☐ Short attention span
☐ Uncontrollable
☐ Sleeping problems
☐ Poor motor coordination
☐ Flares up easily
☐ Disrupts household, playground, classroom

Dr. Feingold's therapy, and eliminate them from their diet. Keeping these foods off their diet, even if your kids don't show symptoms of hyperactivity, can prevent salicylate-induced hyperactivity from ever striking.

But salicylate-food elimination is a harsh measure to take. Practically, it means making one set of menus for your kids and one for you and your husband, and that's a burden. Psychologically, it sets the kids apart and makes them feel freakish, with all the consequent wounds to the ego. Nutritionally, it denies the kids the benefits of foods which, aside from the salicylate content, are bountifully nutritious.

Yet until recently, elimination of salicylates was the only way to prevent and cure salicylate-induced hyperactivity. Now there's a new way based on discoveries, made by dozens of independent medical investigators, that explain how salicylates work in the brain to induce hyperactivity.

What these investigators learned is this: Salicylates sharply re-

Do Your Kids Exhibit Hyperactivity Symptoms After Eating Any of These Foods?

•—————————————•

If they do, the hyperactivity is induced by aspirinlike substances, called salicylates, in the foods. You can then strike all these foods from your kids' meals, or you can switch your kids to our Eating Plan for Brighter Kids. It protects against salicylates, and lets your kids enjoy these tasty and nutritious foods.

Fruits
- ☐ Apples
- ☐ Apricots
- ☐ Blackberries
- ☐ Boysenberries
- ☐ Cherries
- ☐ Currants
- ☐ Gooseberries
- ☐ Grapes
- ☐ Nectarines
- ☐ Oranges
- ☐ Peaches
- ☐ Plums
- ☐ Prunes
- ☐ Raisins
- ☐ Raspberries
- ☐ Strawberries

Vegetables
- ☐ Cucumbers, cucumber pickles
- ☐ Tomatoes, tomato products

duce the amounts of vitamin C in children's brains, as well as vitamins of the B-complex and the minerals calcium, potassium, and iron. Deprivation of *any* of these nutrients may result in hyperactivity, and salicylates cause deprivation of *all* of them.

To offset the effects of salicylate-containing foods *without removing them from your kids' diet*, today's medical nutrition scientists recommend a diet with the *right* high amounts of vitamins and minerals to compensate for the loss of those nutrients due to salicylates.

Because you're likely to find it so difficult to create such a diet that you might throw up your hands in despair, we've tailored that diet *for* you—our Eating Plan for Brighter Kids. What you'll like about this Plan is that there's just one basic menu for the entire family; kids don't feel alienated; and they enjoy nutritious foods that otherwise would be forbidden.

Protecting Your Kids Against Additives

Dr. Feingold found that in some of his patients the elimination of salicylate-rich foods did not remedy hyperactivity. Could there be other substances in foods that produced the disorder? He put two and two together.

Before the 1950s hyperactivity was virtually unknown. But during the 1950s the processed-food industry expanded enormously. Throughout the nation, natural foods were replaced with foods containing additives—chemical colorings, flavorings, preservatives, stimulants, and processing ingredients. Could additives cause hyperactivity?

The first indication that they could came, surprisingly, from an adult patient. Before coming to Dr. Feingold, she had been treated by psychotherapy for years with no success. When Dr. Feingold switched the psychotherapeutic drug she was on to one containing no artificial coloring, she was suddenly cured. If an abnormal emotional/behavioral problem in an adult could be caused by an additive, surely, Dr. Feingold reasoned, it was possible for additives to cause hyperactivity in a child.

Dr. Feingold examined the diets of hyperactive kids who were not cured by salicylate-food elimination. All of those diets contained additives. When Dr. Feingold switched the diets back to natural foods (as Sara Sloan was doing about the same time for her kids, and with similar results), hyperactivity changed back to normality.

Dr. Feingold's therapy for hyperactives, he reported, was spectacularly effective. "Disturbances . . . usually of many years duration [showed] favorable response within days. . . . The child loses his hyperkinesis [hyperactivity], his motor incoordination, and becomes well-adjusted. The sleep pattern improves. Drugs that have been administered for several years can be discontinued."

He added, "Improved scholastic achievement is also dramatic. Within a single quarter at school the child will show much improvement in his reading and writing ability as well as with numbers.

. . . These children [then] have either a normal or a high I.Q."

His notebooks glow with successful cases.

"On July 2nd," one entry reads, "Johnny C. began [my additive-free diet] and on July 8th, a startling six days later, his mother told me, 'He's become very quiet . . . easy to control.' He was able to reason with parents and peers."

But on July 13, the child cheated. He "ate a bakery doughnut at 7 A.M. and by 10 A.M. was hyperactive, unable to use self-control. Twenty-four hours later, after the food had cleared his system, he was back to the 'new normal.' "

In just a few days, and sometimes overnight, kids who had been the bane of their parents' and teachers' lives were suddenly normal —an amazing record for rapidity of cure of a major medical disorder.

So impressed with the speed of Dr. Feingold's results were eminent nutrition scientists Dr. Emanuel Cheraskin and Dr. W. Marshall Ringsdorf that they enthusiastically described the behavior changes of hyperactive kids on an additive-free diet as "like . . . switching a light from 'On' to 'Off.' "

But the parents who cut down, without entirely eliminating, hyperactivity-inducing foods in their kids' diet, found no switch off. The reason, Dr. Feingold discovered after years of persistent investigation, is that the substances in food that activate hyperactivity are effective in extremely small quantities.

"I remain stunned," he wrote years after he made that discovery, "by the infinitesimal amounts of activator [needed] . . . stunned that any substance of 50 trillionth of a gram could react in the human [brain]." To defeat hyperactivity, he told parents, foods that induce it must be banned *entirely*. A list of Dr. Feingold's hyperactivity-inducing foods appears on pages 42–43.

But just a cursory glance at Dr. Feingold's forbidden list is enough to frighten off most mothers. It eliminates virtually all packaged, canned, frozen, prepared, and fast foods; and it puts all but the fresh food departments of the supermarket out of bounds. The strains of extended kitchen-and-shopping time and getting the kids accustomed to new tastes, on top of the burden of preparing one meal for the hyperactive kids and another for the rest of the family, makes acceptance of Dr. Feingold's Spartan regimen difficult to impossible.

That's one reason doctors, realizing that a nonadditives diet is sooner or later rejected, prescribe drugs for hyperactive kids.

But they don't work.

Hyperactive kids are treated mainly with members of a family of drugs called central nervous system stimulants. Paradoxically, these drugs—Ritalin and Cyclert are examples—do not stimulate hyperactive kids as they do other kids and adults, but rather calm them down. But abnormally so—a full pendulum swing.

"These drugs may control impulsive and distracting behavior, but they also turn children into submissive, zombie-like creatures," observes Dr. Allan Cott. "Depression and withdrawal are frequent side effects, and so in the end, the drugs defeat the very purpose for which they are prescribed—to give the child the tranquillity and eagerness to learn."

Other common side effects are also far from conducive to the child's health, happiness, and learning ability. They include: insomnia, loss of appetite, loss of weight, dizziness, nausea, stomachaches, drowsiness, and headaches.

Doctors also prescribe members of the phenothiazine family of drugs—such as Thorazine, Mellaril-S, and chlorpromazine hydrochloride—for some cases of hyperactivity. Originally formulated for use in treatment of psychiatric disorders characterized by psychotic agitation, aggressiveness, and explosive, intense excitability, these drugs are claimed by the manufacturers to be effective on hyperactive kids when used over a short period.

But the side effects can be devastating. Some of them actually accomplish the reverse of what the drugs are supposed to do, producing such symptoms as restlessness, excitement, trembling, shaking hands and fingers, jerky movements of hands and neck, involuntary tongue and mouth movements, and fast heartbeat. Intense drowsiness and sharp decline of mental alertness may result as well, sometimes accompanied by light-headedness, dizziness, and fainting.

"*Drugs resolve no . . . problems,*" writes Dr. Cott, referring to their use in the treatment of hyperactivity and other learning disorders. "*They only disguise symptoms temporarily* (emphasis his)." He points out that drug therapy for children with learning problems including hyperactivity has been banned in Sweden and Japan, commenting that it's "certainly a wise measure."

Additives-Containing Foods That Can Trigger Hyperactivity

• ——————————————— •

Each child has an individual trigger level at which certain amounts of additives can induce hyperactivity. Trigger levels are so low in some children that they're reached by infinitesimal amounts of additives. The best way to prevent your children from reaching these levels is to strike all additives-containing foods from their diet. The additives-containing foods on this list, compiled by Dr. Ben F. Feingold, are included in our 181 Worst Foods for Your Kids' Brains in Chapter 11. Many are replaced in our Eating Plan for Brighter Kids with healthful nonadditive taste-alikes.

Breakfast Cereals

All with artificial colors or flavors
All instant breakfast preparations

Baked Goods

All manufactured baked goods, fresh and frozen, including cakes, cookies, pastry, sweet rolls, pies, doughnuts, and breads
All packaged baking mixes

Luncheon Meats

All packaged meats, including bologna, salami, frankfurters, sausages, meat loaf, bacon, ham, and pork

Poultry

All barbecued and self-basting poultry
All prepared stuffing

Fish

All fish sticks
All artificially dyed or flavored frozen fillets

Desserts

All ice creams, sherbets, and ices
All gelatin and junket desserts
All puddings
All dessert mixes
All flavored yogurts

Candies

All manufactured candies

Beverages

All instant breakfast drinks
All quick-mix powdered drinks
Tea, coffee, and chocolate milk
Soft drinks, including diet drinks

Other Items

All mint-flavored items
All mustards and ketchups
Soy sauces that are artificially flavored or colored,
and chili sauces
Artificially colored butter and margarine
Cider and wine vinegar
Cloves

To dramatize the wide gulf between drug and dietary treatment of hyperactivity, he cites a case described in the *Journal of Orthomolecular Medicine:*

A 12-year-old girl, diagnosed as hyperactive, had been committed to a number of institutions. Treatment consisted of heavy doses of amphetamines "washed down with tumblers of sugar-ridden soft drinks." Amphetamines are central nervous system stimulants, known on the street as "speed" or "uppers." Sugar is a stimulant that acts on hyperactive kids just as it does on anybody else.

When medication was gradually reduced, and finally terminated, "the girl was placed on a diet free of junk food," Dr. Cott reports, "and within weeks . . . her hyperactivity disappeared. With improved motor coordination, she learned how to run and swim. Her intellectual performance rose steadily.

"Without dietary control," Dr. Cott concludes, *"there is no doubt that she would have remained on medication and in an institution for the rest of her life* (emphasis ours)."

But with drugs useless and harmful, and with an additives-free diet presenting onerous practical difficulties, there seems to be no viable way to fight additives-induced hyperactivity.

That's one reason we created our Eating Plan for Brighter Kids— to provide such a way for you.

It supplies additives-free menus you can prepare with minimum kitchen-and-shopping time.

It presents no taste barrier, because it includes some "rehabilitated" junk foods, processed foods once additives-packed but now free of additives; and our healthful "junk-food clones" that taste and even look like the additives kind.

It can be enjoyed by the whole family; so you never have to make one meal for your kids and another for yourself and your husband.

Dr. Bernard Rimland, Director of the Institute for Child Behavior Research in San Diego, affirmed in 1986 that "it is quite well established . . . that Feingold was in fact correct . . . and [that] a large number of hyperactive children can be controlled by [his] diet." Our Eating Plan for Brighter Kids is, among other things, a simple drug-free program to fight hyperactivity the Feingold way—without the drawbacks of the Feingold diet.

• CHAPTER •
3

"CEREBRAL ALLERGENS"

Foods That Could Make Your Kids
Slow Learners

The 1950s saw the epidemic rise of learning disabilities, not yet abated, of which hyperactivity is one major cause. There's another, the opposite of hyperactivity: the slow-learning syndrome. Its mental symptoms are fatigue, drowsiness, depression, anxiety, and a feeling of tension, always accompanied by slow learning.

Puzzled by this syndrome—which was not then effectively treated (as it still is not today) by therapeutic drugs, psychiatry, or counseling—pediatrician Dr. William G. Crook, following Dr. Feingold's lead, looked for the foods that cause it.

After about 20 years of clinical research, which incorporated the results of other investigators, he found them. In 1973, he introduced to an astonished general public a new class of foods that could affect kids adversely—cerebral allergens. They are so called, he said, because they have an allergic effect on kids' brains.

Are Your Kids Slow Learners Because of Cerebral Allergens?

Dr. Crook discovered a simple way for you to find out. Cerebral allergens, he learned, are likely to be the cause of slow learning when the complete slow-learning syndrome is accompanied by at least a few of the following physical symptoms:

Physical Symptoms That May Accompany the Slow-Learning Syndrome
• ——————————— •

- [ ] Paleness
- [ ] Feeling blah
- [ ] Circles or bags under eyes
- [ ] Stuffy nose
- [ ] Sinus complaints
- [ ] Excessive sneezing
- [ ] Belly aches
- [ ] Muscle pains

- [ ] Itching
- [ ] Rashes
- [ ] Bedwetting or other urinary problems
- [ ] Headaches
- [ ] Puffiness or bloating
- [ ] Coughing or wheezing
- [ ] Chest discomfort

If a kid of yours *is* a slow learner because of cerebral allergens, then one or more of the following foods may be responsible.

The Slow-Learning Foods
• ——————————— •

- [ ] Beans, particularly soybeans
- [ ] Breads and other baked goods
- [ ] Breakfast cereals
- [ ] Corn and corn products such as corn oil and tacos
- [ ] Grapefruit
- [ ] Lemons
- [ ] Lentils
- [ ] Limes
- [ ] Malted milks

- [ ] Oranges
- [ ] Pancakes
- [ ] Peanuts
- [ ] Peas
- [ ] Potatoes
- [ ] Soy sauce
- [ ] Stuffings
- [ ] Tofu (bean curd)
- [ ] Waffles
- [ ] Wheat germ

But *which* of these cerebral allergens affects *your* child? Dr. Crook has discovered that a cerebral allergen that triggers the total slow-learning syndrome (physical and mental symptoms) in one child, need not be the one that triggers it in another. To pinpoint the specific cerebral allergens affecting your child, Dr. Crook pioneered a method now recommended, with variations, by many physicians:

- You feed your child an "elimination diet" that leaves out one possible cerebral allergen for seven to eight days.

- Should the symptoms of the total slow-learning syndrome improve for two days, then you've found a "suspect food."

- You then return the suspect food to your child's diet; and if after about a week all the symptoms return in full strength, you know the suspect food is a "guilty food"—a cerebral allergen.

- The food is then permanently eliminated from the child's diet.

- When it is, or when several cerebral allergens discovered in the same way are eliminated, your slow-learning child's life can be turned around, Dr. Crook reports.

Arlene, who is a composite of the thousands of slow learners who have been treated at The Children's Clinic in Jackson, Tennessee, headed by Dr. Crook, was an unhappy, disturbed child who had lost confidence in herself when she became Dr. Crook's patient.

The fifth-grader was behind all the other kids in her class. The other kids made fun of her, and she was sure her teacher hated her. Actually, her teacher was trying to help when she scolded Arlene and gave her bad grades, but it just made the child think worse of herself. The teacher would say, "Arlene, you're really a *smart* girl. You could do better if you really *wanted* to and *tried*." But Arlene would complain to Dr. Crook, "I *want* to but I *can't*. Why *should* I try?"

Dr. Crook's elimination diet pinpointed Arlene's cerebral allergens. When they were removed from her diet, within weeks she seemed to her parents to be a "new child."

"She felt better," Dr. Crook observed. "She performed better in school, and when she performed better, she received praise and her self-esteem increased. This, in turn, caused her to try harder. . . . As a result of all these things working together, her learning problems . . . improved or disappeared [and so did] her emotional problems."

Other doctors using Dr. Crook's therapy reported similar successes. One task force of pediatric clinicians headed by Dr. William C. Deamer of the University of California, San Francisco, in a paper which appeared in the prestigious scientific journal *Pediatrics*, compared standard medical treatment of slow-learning kids with Dr. Crook's method:

"During the last several years we've seen 94 children with . . . syndromes caused by [cerebral] allergy who previously had been treated by conventional doctors. [Some of these kids] had been investigated for brain tumors . . . studied for anemia . . . and referred to psychiatrists because of their behavior."

There had been no improvement in their conditions. But when Dr. Deamer's pediatric task force eliminated brain allergens in the kids' diets, "the symptoms [of slow learning] improved or disappeared."

The task force recommended to fellow pediatricians that "patients with similar symptoms be given the benefit of an elimination diet before attributing their symptoms to [other than nutritional] causes."

But Dr. Crook's cerebral allergen treatment, as sound and effective as it is, has several practical drawbacks.

Most elimination-diet searches for specific cerebral allergens are not as simple as they appear to be. Many foods may have to undergo the elimination test before a guilty food is found. Often many guilty foods are involved, and then the search becomes complex and prolonged, and must be undertaken under medical supervision. Doctors' fees, time, and tension mount.

Besides, mothers found—as other mothers had found when their kids had been put on Dr. Feingold's additives-free diet—that a special diet for one or more kids in the family creates problems. Preparing two meals, one for the afflicted kids, and the other for the rest of the family, is a grueling chore. Kids resent having to give up foods they've become accustomed to. Parents worry about their kids missing the nutrients in the banned foods.

Parents told Dr. Crook that the elimination diet is worth all the dollar, time, and emotional costs involved, but they wished there was an easier way.

There is—now.

It's based on the recent discoveries of medical allergy specialists and medical nutrition scientists concerning Dr. Crook's cerebral allergens.

The New Way to Feed
Slow-Learning Kids to Brightness

The first discovery is that cerebral allergens are not allergens.

To Dr. Crook, an allergy is "a hypersensitivity to a specific substance which, in similar quantity, does not bother other people." That "specific substance" is an allergen.

Not necessarily so, respond medical allergy specialists. For a substance to be an allergen, it must react with antibodies (proteins normally necessary to the body's defense against disease) to create a harmful reaction—an allergic reaction.

Only a laboratory test, these specialists assert, can determine whether a substance reacts harmfully with antibodies, and is indeed an allergen. They found that Dr. Crook's list of cerebral allergens that passed his elimination test could not pass their laboratory test. The foods that Dr. Crook had identified as causing slow-learning kids were not allergens.

Actually, Dr. Crook didn't know what they were. He had adopted the term *allergen* because when he began his research allergy was a medical fad, and doctors were diagnosing symptoms they didn't understand as an "allergy" (as now they're diagnosing them as a "virus"). But of one thing Dr. Crook was certain: The foods he had identified *did* cause the total slow-learning syndrome.

Today's medical nutrition scientists agree, but their research points to a new explanation of how these foods may act on kids' brains. What appears to happen is this:

The cerebral allergens diminish the brain's supply of certain vitamins and minerals to below the levels that prevent the total slow-learning syndrome. Those levels are different for every child, which explains why some kids are affected and some are not.

The minerals include calcium, copper, iron, magnesium, phosphorus, zinc, selenium and chromium. Among the vitamins are vitamin C, and those of the B-complex, especially B_6 and pantothenic acid. There is good evidence that many of those nutrients help protect as well against allergens other than cerebral.

Nutrition scientists point out that when the quantities of the vitamins and minerals lost to kids' brains by the action of cerebral allergens are replenished by a diet high in those nutrients, the cerebral allergens need not be removed from kids' diets. One study demonstrated that on this type of diet, I.Q.'s rapidly soared up to 35 points; and in another study, reading scores swiftly leaped up to 3.4 grade levels.

The chances are you'll find it difficult to create a diet with just the right amounts of the vitamins and minerals your kids need to fight cerebral allergens. Too little would be ineffective; too much would be dangerous.

Our Eating Plan for Brighter Kids resolves that difficulty for you by providing the optimal amounts of vitamins and minerals to help protect your child against the slow-learning syndrome.

• CHAPTER •

4

SUGAR

Foods That Could Turn Your Kids into Jekyll-and-Hydes

The world's most popular sweetener is pure, white, crystalline sucrose—sugar.

This is a sampling from the indictment against it as an enemy of kids' brains:

At Eunice Moss' Richard Forrest School in Virginia, winsome 7-year-olds who scored consistent A's in reading during the morning, after a sugary lunch became bad-tempered and couldn't even recognize the letters of the alphabet.

Dr. Hugh L. Powers, a pediatrician working with the Dallas school system, was appalled to discover that too many kids in all grades following heavy sugar lunches sank into depression, anxiety, gloom, lethargy, and just plain feeling rotten. These are "sugar-blues" kids whose learning disabilities can be as severe as hyperactives'.

Anxious mothers complain to doctors that their normal kids "climb the walls" after birthdays, holidays, and trick-or-treat time —that is, after they've gorged themselves with sugar-packed candies, cakes, and ice creams.

Doctors' records are replete with cases of well-behaved kids who suddenly explode with anger, go into temper tantrums, and flare into irrational outbursts following sugar-filled meals.

A study at the American Institute of Biosocial Research, Jacksonville Beach, Florida, conducted by Alexander C. Schauss, linked the onset of learning disabilities to a high-sugar diet, and found that when the diet was continued, nine out of ten of the learning-disabled kids developed into juvenile delinquents.

51

When Dr. Stephen J. Schoenthaler, coordinator of the criminal justice research program at California State University, Turlock, switched juvenile delinquents in 17 correction institutions and 803 schools to a low- or no-sugar diet, he found he could "reduce by half antisocial behavior like assault, theft and insubordination."

Dr. Sidney W. Mintz, a professor at Johns Hopkins University, who is an expert on foods that also are drugs, explains the swift changes in behavior induced by being "on" or "off" sugar by identifying sugar as a mind-altering drug.

What all this evidence, and much more like it, demonstrates dramatically is at bottom a simple fact: Many kids on high-sugar meals are Hydes, and on low-sugar meals become Jekylls and vice versa.

Can You Keep Sugar in Your Kids' Diet?

No. These are the reasons:

Sugar, because it stimulates the flow of insulin, depresses the amount of glucose in your child's bloodstream. Not enough glucose, the brain's source of energy, is carried to the brain. Among the many symptoms of low glucose are: irritability, loss of concentration and attention, faltering memory, depression, anxiety, light-headedness, dizziness, insomnia, fatigue, and exhaustion.

Even in the mildest cases of this sugar-induced disorder, Dr. Allan Cott observes, "The brain function . . . is impaired. Even if [a child] does not suffer from a learning disability, he will not learn as well as he should."

The simplest, safest, and the only effective way to prevent or reverse sugar-induced low-glucose symptoms is to eliminate dietary sugar.

Sugar leads to physical disorders as well. Dr. John Yudkin, the leading British pioneer among medical nutrition scientists, in his aptly entitled book *Pure, White and Deadly*, associates the sweetener with an astonishing spectrum of diseases. They include obesity, diabetes, gout, atherosclerosis, heart attack, enlargement of the liver, kidney damage, chronic indigestion, gastric and duodenal ulcers, and dental decay.

There's no way to prevent sugar's contribution to the onset of these diseases except by removing the sweetener from your kids' menus.

Sugar also undernourishes your children even though it seems that they're well fed. Here's what happens:

If your child's diet is like the diet of most American children, it's 50 percent sugar in terms of total calories. Sugar is an "empty-calorie" food—a food that contributes calories (energy) but no, or virtually no, vitamins and minerals. Subtract 50 percent of sugar's empty calories from the, say, 1,200 calories each of your children consumes daily, and that leaves 600 calories a day of nutritious foods (provided all the nonsugar foods are nutritious, which they're probably not). That's undernourishment.

In addition to curtailing growth and weakening your child's resistance to disease, undernourishment produces these symptoms: lack of concentration, memory loss, irritability, depression, and inability to think clearly.

The child who exhibits these symptoms—it could be your child—is not alone. According to the *Bulletin of the Foundation for Nutrition and Stress Research,* out of every 1,000 American kids, 999 are victims of some degree of undernourishment. One out of every three American kids, the National Nutrition Survey conducted by the U.S. Department of Human Services adds, exhibits symptoms of *severe* undernourishment.

Sugar has also led to a strange new kind of American tragedy, according to Dr. Bernard Rimland. Obnoxious personality traits in our children resulting from sugar-induced vitamin and mineral deficiencies, he states, have become so widespread that they are now regarded as the norm for growing up in America.

Sugar, for all these reasons, is regarded by forefront medical opinion as the ingredient in the American diet most dangerous to kids.

Cutting down on sugar, unless you cut it down to almost zero, won't help, because you'll still be feeding your kids empty calories at a time when their growing bodies and brains need *all* the required number of nutritious calories. The only *sure* way to avoid sugar-induced undernourishment is to cut out sugar *entirely* from their diet.

Says Dr. Allan Cott: "I applaud the mother who told me she painted a skull and crossbones on the sugar canister in her home."

Can You Use Sugar Substitutes?

Yes and no. Many sugar substitutes are also empty-calorie foods; and other substitutes are disqualified for other health reasons. But some substitutes are excellent. Let the list on pages 55–57 be your guide. It was ours when we prepared our Eating Plan for Brighter Kids.

But aren't kids born with a taste for sugar—real sugar?

If that's so, then kids have been deprived for all but a few of the many long years that the human race has been on earth. Sugar did not become a people's food until little more than a hundred years ago when it was introduced in England as a stimulant (in tea, another stimulant) to fight off exhaustion among the men, women, *and* children who toiled for twelve to sixteen hours without breaks in Britain's mills and factories. The use of sugar then spread throughout the industrial West, and then to the world.

Nowhere in the scientific literature is there any evidence that kids are born with a taste for sugar. Dr. Allan Cott states flatly, "No baby is born with a sweet tooth. A child will not clamor for more cookies, unless that child has been fed cookies. The taste for [sugar] is acquired."

Easily acquired. But, as every health-conscious mother knows, hard to break. Until now.

How to Break Your Kids' Sugar Habit

It's smart to start by banning sugar in your kitchen—out of sight is out of mouth—but the real danger doesn't come from the sugar you can see; it comes from the sugar you can't see.

The more than half pound of sugar daily (and rising) that average American adults consume doesn't come from the sugar they spoon into their tea or coffee, but from the sugar hidden in virtually all junk foods. Sugar is insidiously omnipresent in soft drinks; chocolates; pies; cookies; Jell-O; puddings; jams and jellies; all yogurts except plain; baking mixes; breads; breakfast cereals; ketchup and other condiments; and even in canned, frozen, and packaged meats, poultry, fish, fruits, and vegetables.

A Parent's Guide to Sugar Substitutes

Substitute	Guideline	Comments
Aspartame	Do not use.	See EQUAL.
Beet sugar (raw, unrefined; 96 percent SUCROSE)	Do not use.	Empty-calorie food.
Blackstrap molasses (96 percent SUCROSE)	Do not use.	Empty-calorie food.
Brown sugar (sucrose plus a small quantity of molasses)	Do not use.	Empty-calorie food.
Cane sugar (raw, unrefined; 96 percent SUCROSE)	Do not use.	Empty-calorie food.
Carrot juice	Okay to use, but see comments.	Excessive use may result in liver damage to susceptible kids (and adults).
Coconut	Use sparingly.	Good supply of nutrients, but high in saturated fat, which can be harmful in excess.
Corn syrup (an invert-type sugar; see INVERT SUGAR)	Do not use.	Empty-calorie food.
Date powder (crushed dried dates)	Okay to use.	Good supply of nutrients.
Date sugar (same as DATE POWDER)	Okay to use.	Good supply of nutrients.
Dextrins (chemical relatives of DEXTROSE)	Do not use.	Empty-calorie food.
Dextrose (a form of GLUCOSE)	Do not use	Empty-calorie food.
Dried fruits (raisins, dates, apples, bananas, etc.)	Okay to use.	Good supply of nutrients.
Equal (active ingredients are ASPARTAME, DEXTROSE, and dried CORN SYRUP)	Do not use.	Empty-calorie food; harmful to kids with phenylketonuria, a brain disorder.
Fructose (refined fruit sugar)	Do not use.	Empty-calorie food.
Fruit (raw or cooked without sugar)	Okay to use.	Good supply of nutrients.
Fruit juices (fresh or frozen concentrates)	Okay to use.	Good supply of nutrients; fresh is better.

A Parent's Guide to Sugar Substitutes (cont.)

Substitute	Guideline	Comments
Fruit pastes (no sugar or salt added)	Okay to use.	Good supply of nutrients.
Glucose (a form of DEXTROSE)	Do not use.	Empty-calorie food.
Herbs (sweet: such as aniseed, marjoram, oregano, rosemary, sweet basil, and tarragon)	Okay to use.	Good supply of nutrients.
HFCS (high-FRUCTOSE CORN SYRUP)	Do not use.	Empty-calorie food.
Honey (raw, unfiltered, uncooked)	Okay to use, but see comments.	Good supply of nutrients, *but do not use* for children under age 1 (raw honey has been implicated in infant deaths), and *do not use* if honey has been made from the nectar of the following plants: azalea, mountain laurel, yellow jasmine, and some rhododendrons. These honeys may be toxic.
Honey (processed)	Do not use.	Much of the nutrient value has been destroyed in processing.
Invert sugar (a mixture of roughly equal amounts of FRUCTOSE and GLUCOSE)	Do not use.	Empty-calorie food.
Mannitol (a sugarlike substance)	Do not use.	Empty-calorie food.
Maple syrup (100 percent pure, untreated)	Use sparingly, but see comments.	Low nutrient value, due to extraction process; but *do not use* unless label states no toxic formaldehyde insecticide has been employed on the trees (the insecticide is banned by law in Canada).

56

Maple syrup (commercial, a mixture of CORN and SUCROSE SYRUPS plus artificial coloring, with little MAPLE SYRUP)	Do not use.	Empty-calorie food, worsened by artificial coloring.
Nut pastes (no sugar or salt added)	Okay to use.	Good supply of nutrients.
NutraSweet (essential ingredient is ASPARTAME; see EQUAL)	Do not use.	See EQUAL.
Nuts (raw)	Okay to use.	Good supply of nutrients.
Pancake syrups (see MAPLE SYRUP, commercial)	Do not use.	See MAPLE SYRUP, commercial.
Raw sugar (96 percent SUCROSE with a small amount of molasses)	Do not use.	Empty-calorie food.
Saccharin	Do not use.	Possible carcinogen.
Sorbitol (a sugarlike substance)	Do not use.	Empty-calorie food.
Spices (sweet: such as allspice, cinnamon, coriander, ginger, mace, and mild paprika)	Okay to use.	Good supply of nutrients
Sugar cane	Okay to use.	Good supply of nutrients.
Turbinado sugar (96 percent SUCROSE with a small amount of molasses)	Do not use.	Empty-calorie food.
Yellow-D (96 percent SUCROSE with a small amount of molasses)	Do not use.	Empty-calorie food.
Xylitol (a sugarlike substance)	Do not use.	Empty-calorie food.

The New "Super-Sweeteners": Thaumatin, derived from the West African kafemfe bush, is the sweetest substance known to science—100,000 times sweeter than sugar. Monellin, which comes from the serendipity berry of another African bush, is almost as sweet. Little is known as yet about their effects on humans. Levo-O-Cal, a "left-handed" version of sucrose, has no nutritive value at all, not even caloric value, because it cannot be metabolized by the body. None of these new super-sweeteners is yet available commercially.

Shockingly, sugar in kids' diets is even higher than adults—by 25 percentage points. The blame for that rests with TV-hustled "kids' foods"—breakfast cereals, soft drinks, snacks, desserts, frozen dinners, and fast food—all junk foods glutted with sugar.

So, breaking the sugar habit really means breaking the junk-food habit. That's why we've created *healthful* "junk-food clones"—especially desserts and snacks—to replace sugar-heavy junk foods.

There are two kinds of our healthful junk foods, both deliciously sweetened with sugar-free sweeteners. One does not contain a single grain of sugar. The other contains negligible amounts of sugar. (There's no harm done by a few empty calories, because the nutrient loss is made up on our high vitamin/mineral diet.)

The slightly sugared junk foods help your kids make the transition to sugar-free junk foods in this way:

Children may not take to the taste of the sugar-free clones at once; there *is* a taste difference. But the difference is not appreciable, and after a while when you introduce the sugar-free junk-food clones, your children won't taste too much difference, and will get used to them easily and enjoyably. Your kids will have acquired a new taste. Then you can drop the slightly sugared junk foods—and all real junk foods, and all sugar—from your children's menus forever.

And from yours and your husband's, too, when you make the same transition. Sugar is as bad for adults—bringing on sugar blues, threatening health with nutrition scientist Dr. Yudkin's long catalog of sugar-induced diseases, and playing havoc with hopes of slimness. Yet when you and the rest of the family switch over to nonsugar foods our healthful junk-food way, your sweet tooth will be as satisfied as it was before. This is a sweet way to break the sugar habit.

You'll find a list of our healthful "junk-food clones" in Chapter 13.

• CHAPTER •
5

IODINE AND GOITROGENS

Foods That Could Slash Your Kids' I.Q.'s

Watch for this combination of symptoms in your kids:

Swelling in the neck below the chin. Loss of muscular coordination, especially finger coordination. Depression. Sudden outbursts of anger over trifles. Hostility. Extreme slowness in walking, talking, eating, playing—in doing anything. Fatigue. And most of all, a precipitate decline in mental activity.

These are symptoms of a disease that had been virtually wiped out in the United States, but is now returning. In its preliminary stages—no perceptible swelling, all the symptoms mild—about 20 million Americans are already affected, estimates Dr. Michael Colgan. Children are its particular victims. The disease is goiter.

The return of goiter is the result, paradoxically, of two recent changes in the American way of eating widely hailed as beneficial: less salt, and a greater variety of natural foods in our diet. Here's how those changes for the better can worsen your kids' I.Q.'s through inducing goiter—and what you can do to prevent it.

How to Protect Your Kids from Goiter—Even on a Low-Salt Diet

Goiter is an iodine-deprivation disease. Iodine is a "trace mineral," a nutrient utilized by the body in infinitesimal quantities. The U.S. Recommended Dietary Allowance (RDA) is 40 to 120 micrograms for children up to age 10, and 150 micrograms for older children and

59

adults. A microgram is one millionth of a gram, or about a twenty-eighth millionth of an ounce.

Consumption of less than the RDA of iodine can induce goiter. That happens when the soil of a region is so poor in iodine that the plant food growing from it, and the livestock nurtured on the plant food, contain little or no iodine. Our Midwest is such a region— "the goiter belt"; and its food, consumed locally, and shipped nationally, once produced an epidemic of goiter.

But since the 1850s, goiter has been almost nonexistent in this country due to a marvel of American ingenuity: iodine added to table salt—iodized salt. Only a sixth of a teaspoon of iodized salt in a day can prevent your kids from ever coming down with goiter induced by iodine deficiency; and most of the salt in the USA is iodized.

But in recent years salt has gone out of fashion. The milestone discovery made by nutrition scientists in the 1950s that excess salt may be responsible in some cases for high blood pressure (hypertension), the "silent killer" associated with a catalog of deadly diseases including heart attack and kidney disorders, has become official medical dogma. Pediatricians, alert now to the dangers of hypertension, include blood pressure measurement in routine examinations, and their findings are frightening: Hypertension is common even among preschool children.

Less salt is often prescribed. Some doctors go so far as banning salt entirely, explaining that children can get their RDA of sodium (the major component of salt) from the foods on the average American diet. But in their rush—a laudable one—to protect children from hypertension, they've overlooked this ugly fact: The average American diet is short in iodine. And the sodium (salt) in it is not iodized. Some doctors now fear that padlocking the salt shaker means swapping hypertension for goiter.

This puts you, as it does all the parents in America, in a quandary. How can you lower your kids' iodized salt intake, and still protect against goiter?

One way is to add iodine to your kids' diet as a component of a mineral supplement. But that presents a new problem: How much shall you add? Too little won't help; and too much iodine can induce the disease it's intended to cure (this is called the Wolff-Chaikoff effect after the doctors who discovered it). In addition, one distressing side effect of iodine overdose is acne.

The hazard-free way to protect your kids from hypertension and goiter simultaneously is to prepare a diet truly low in salt (less than a sixth of a teaspoon added daily) but with just the right amount of iodine—from the foods, the added iodized salt, and a mineral supplement—to ward off goiter.

This diet *is* difficult to create. But don't throw up your hands. This is the diet we've prepared *for* your kids and your whole family (adults, too, need protection against hypertension and goiter) on our Eating Plan for Brighter Kids.

Don't minimize the danger of goiter. Without that trace of iodine, more than 120 million kids throughout the world, mostly in Third World countries, suffer from it. To observe what goiter can do, come with a UNICEF observer to one of the many villages in northern India where goiter is raging. (UNICEF is the acronym for the United Nations' Children's Fund.) But be warned by the observer: "Walking into these villages is absolutely mind-shattering."

Look at the children. There are growths under their chins, grotesque, as big as eggs. In some kids, they're as enormous as softballs. Ordinary things children do—walking, eating, talking—are performed in zombielike slow motion. The kids are freakishly awkward, shambling, disoriented. Finger coordination is all but gone. Picking up a pebble is a long, laborious, monumental achievement. Weaving a needle and thread through cloth is a frustrating impossibility.

You're in a village where the kids—all of them—are unmistakably dead tired, eyes blank with depression. The slightest change—a fly alighting on a hand—triggers a hot flash of irritation. As they look at each other, at the adults, at you, their hostility is tangible. Talk to them and you'll be appalled by their abysmal mental incapacity. What you tell them, they forget in minutes. Some of the kids have I.Q.'s as low as 20.

The generally milder goiter here—and in Canada and other Western countries—does not stem mainly from an impoverished, low-to no-iodine diet, as it does in Third World countries. Rather it arises from our affluent varied diet which now contains certain dangerous foods, many of which only fairly recently have become supermarket staples. These foods attack the iodine in your kids' bodies and induce goiter. These are the goitrogens.

How to Protect Your Kids from Natural Foods That Trigger Goiter

In recent years goiter struck 33 percent of the kids in Richmond County, Virginia; 42 percent of the kids in Western Columbia, Canada; and 58 percent of the kids in regions throughout the Western world. There is no doubt to Dr. Josef Matovinovic, professor of Internal Medicine, University of Michigan Medical School, and perhaps the nation's leading authority on goitrogens, that "The natural goitrogens in feed and food [were] the significant determinants in [the] prevalence and severity of . . . goiter."

These natural goitrogens attack iodine in the thyroid, a gland in the neck below the chin (its swelling is the blatant symptom of goiter). With insufficient iodine, this gland cannot manufacture thyroxine, a hormone that manages the transport of blood to the brain. With a faltering supply of blood, the brain operates at only a small percentage of its capacity. In addition, lack of thyroxine has a direct adverse effect on brain cells (neurons) and on the biochemicals that make the brain work (the neurotransmitters). The result, the same as from iodine-deprivation caused by iodine-deficient foods, is goiter.

There's a list of natural goitrogens on page 63. It's your guide to which goitrogens to strike off your kids' menus forever, and to which goitrogens are safe to use under certain conditions.

In protecting your kids from goitrogens, here's what to keep in mind:

Each child has an individual trigger level for each goitrogen—the amount of a goitrogen needed before it can attack the iodine in the thyroid. Some children's trigger levels may be so high that the kids cannot be affected by amounts of goitrogens in normal servings. But since you don't know your child's trigger levels—and currently there's no way medical science can tell you—it's best to treat every goitrogen as a potential danger, and take these precautions:

A diet supplying the RDA for iodine will not counteract the depletion of iodine by some goitrogens. But a diet with higher than RDA amounts—ODA amounts, Optimal Dietary Allowances—will. Such a diet is provided for you on our Eating Plan for Brighter Kids. It permits you to include such otherwise nutritious goitrogens in the whole family's meals as peanuts, soybeans, and Brussels sprouts.

Natural Food Goitrogens: They Could Lower Your Kids' I.Q.'s

• ———————————— •

The Dangerous Natural-Food Goitrogens

There is no way to counteract these goitrogens among susceptible children, since the addition of iodine to the diet does not
relieve the goitrogenic effects.

> Cabbage (raw)
> Mustard greens
> Piñon (female seed-pine) nuts
> Rape.

The "Safe" Natural-Food Goitrogens

Addition of ample iodine to the diet or, in some cases, cooking
neutralizes these otherwise nutritious as well as healthful
foods. (The American Cancer Society, for example, advises frequent servings of Brussels sprouts, cabbage and cauliflower to
help prevent cancer.)

> Beets (when cooked)
> Brussels sprouts
> Cabbage (when cooked)
> Cassava
> Cauliflower
> Horseradish
> Kale
> Peanuts
> Rutabaga
> Soybeans
> Spinach (when cooked)
> Turnips (when cooked)
> Walnuts, Persian
> Watercress

While it's healthy-trendy to serve vegetables raw to prevent loss of nutrients due to cooking, when you serve *these* vegetables raw to your kids, you're serving them goitrogens: beets, cabbage, spinach, and turnips. Cooked, though, these otherwise nutritious foods cease to be goitrogens. (Raw vegetable salads are safe when free of goitrogens.)

Three goitrogens—mustard greens, piñon (female seed-pine) nuts, and rape—are the most dangerous. Their active ingredients are thioglucosides, kinds of sugars, which cannot be neutralized by cooking or iodine supplements. The only way to deal with these goitrogens, which appear on our list of The 181 Worst Foods for Your Kids' Brains in Chapter 11, is to eliminate them from your kids' diet.

But sometimes identifying some of the most dangerous goitrogens is difficult, because they're "hidden" in apparently safe foods. Cabbage, rape, and mustard greens are a major source of animal feed, and you have no way of knowing whether the meat and poultry you serve your kids are contaminated with them. We recommend range-fed animals. One hidden goitrogen, though, is easily spotted if you know the code words on the label. They are PURIFIED PROTEINS, and they conceal that the ingredient has been made with rapeseed meal. No purified-protein products are permitted on our Eating Plan for Brighter Kids.

There are several nonfood synthetic goitrogens as well, but these are ineffective against an ODA-iodine diet, such as the one provided by our Eating Plan for Brighter Kids. They are: the insecticides DDD, DDT, and dieldrin; the pesticide PCB; the fire-retardant PPB; and, perhaps, the fungicide EBDC.

"Prevention of effects of natural and synthetic goitrogens," advises Dr. Josef Matovinovic, should be a continuing public health goal." Our Eating Plan for Brighter Kids is an effective step toward that goal.

· CHAPTER ·
6

ANTI-VITAMIN, ANTI-MINERAL FOODS

Foods That Could Brown Out
Your Kids' Brains

Case History: Sandy, age 10

Major Symptom: Impaired sense perceptions

Diagnosis: Preclinical pellagra

Possible Cause: Breakfast cereals, particularly of the granola type; corn and most corn products; seeds; and vegetable greens

A preclinical disorder is characterized by preliminary symptoms of a disease. Preclinical pellagra is a disorder that affects your kids' brains. A little more than a decade ago, although kids had begun to suffer from it nationwide since the 1950s, it was not a disorder recognized by the medical profession. As a matter of fact, up to that time, the nation's doctors did not believe that such a thing as a preclinical disorder existed.

But once preclinical pellagra was discovered by the then obscure pediatrician Dr. Glen Green in the course of his treatment of Sandy, medical nutrition scientists rapidly identified several dozen more preclinical disorders. They all have this in common: The diseases they precede so severely impair the brain's function, that brightness is blacked out. The preclinical disorder, less severe, browns out kids' brains.

There is no cause now, though, to be concerned about their browning out your kids' brains. The path-breaking therapy that Dr. Green innovated when he treated Sandy, refined by other medical nutrition scientists, is the basis of today's simple way you can protect your kids from virtually all preclinical disorders. This is how Dr. Green treated Sandy:

A year before Sandy became a patient of Dr. Green, the child had loved school and friends and parents and music, and the fun of being a child, had played the piano joyously, and was happy and healthy and bright. But suddenly, Dr. Green said in a speech he would later give before the American Schizophrenic Association, Sandy had suffered an appalling personality change. Complaining of stomach pains and headaches, she had become cranky and irritable, found the piano repulsive, and had sunk to the bottom of her class.

Worst of all, Dr. Green said, were Sandy's impaired sense perceptions. Working from notes made during Dr. Green's speech, medical reporters Ruth Adams and Frank Murray, described them:

"Words on a blackboard look like . . . they wriggle around and move back and forth. There is a fog between her eyes and the blackboard. When she looks in the mirror her face becomes larger, then smaller. Other people's faces seem to do the same. The ground moves between her feet and buildings appear to be falling on her. She sometimes feels she is not really walking on the ground. She hears voices calling her name. She is afraid of the dark, afraid of school, unhappy and depressed."

Standard therapy in the mid-1970s for a patient with Sandy's symptoms was primarily psychiatric care often accompanied by mind-altering drugs—a course of treatment that usually required years, carried the risk of drug dependence, and had an unimpressive record of success. Yet pediatricians of that time faced with Sandy's symptoms would sooner or later have referred her to a child psychiatrist. Dr. Green did not.

In a flash of brilliant insight, he saw Sandy's syndrome as a mix of symptoms that could develop into one of the most dreaded mental diseases known to medical science. It's a disease characterized by severe headaches, intense nervousness, memory loss, and depression, and in its terminal stage by hallucinations and dementia —a world, seen through the victim's eyes, that's bizarre, unstable, unreal—the kind of a world Sandy was beginning to see.

To Dr. Green, Sandy was exhibiting preliminary symptoms— "preclinical symptoms"—of that disease. It's pellagra, and it's caused by the depletion of vitamin B_3 (niacin) in kids' brains. Dr. Green started immediate treatments with vitamin-B_3 supplements in quantities far exceeding the RDA.

"Within two weeks," Dr. Green told the American Schizophrenic

Association, as reported by Adams and Murray, "[Sandy] was greatly improved but still had some complaints. By the end of the month she was completely cured, and returned to her happy, bright, alert self."

On the lookout for preclinical pellagra among his patients, Dr. Green found that one out of ten children was afflicted by it. Large over-RDA doses of vitamin B_3 was the cure; and when a child had been afflicted for only a short time before treatment began, it was a fast cure, restoring the child to health in a few days, and sometimes overnight.

Why did Dr. Green prescribe appreciably more vitamin B_3 than the RDA?

RDAs are Recommended Dietary Allowances, calculated by the Food and Nutrition Board, National Academy of Sciences–National Research Council to prevent the onset in most people of nutrition-deprivation diseases, such as pellagra. These allowances are not sufficient, however, to ward off preclinical symptoms of those diseases in many kids and adults.

The allowances of nutrients necessary to do that are called ODAs, Optimal Dietary Allowances. It was Dr. Green's success with over-RDA dosages of vitamin B_3 that clued medical nutrition scientists to establish ODAs for all vitamins and minerals. ODAs are essential to help protect against preclinical symptoms; that's why your kids get their full ODAs of vitamin B_3, and all other vitamins and minerals, on our Eating Plan for Brighter Kids.

There are several reasons for the amounts of a vitamin or mineral in the brain to fall below its ODA level. But when the deficiency appears suddenly in well-nourished kids—as it did in Sandy's case—medical nutrition scientists look for special kinds of foods newly added to the kids' diets. These are foods that diminish the quantities of certain vitamins and minerals in the brain—the anti-vitamin, anti-mineral foods.

Records of medical nutrition scientists show that as the American diet has changed over the last decade or so, the following anti-vitamin-B_3 foods have made abrupt debuts on the diets of thousands of Sandys:

Some "health foods": seeds, vegetable greens, and raw grains, particularly in granola-type breakfast cereal.

Tex-Mex foods based on corn, including tacos, tortillas, enchiladas, tostadas, and tamales. (Corn may not be a direct vitamin-B_3

antagonist, but it is low in that vitamin as well as in the amino acid tryptophan from which the body manufactures it. The result is vitamin-B₃ deprivation on a diet mainly of corn or most corn products. Corn oil, though, is not an anti-vitamin-B₃ food.)

Successful treatment of preclinical pellagra, from Dr. Green on, never required the removal of the offending but otherwise nutritious foods from the diet. Rather, the contents of vitamin B₃ in kids' brains were brought up to ODA level, and kept there through supplementation. Supplementation cannot be discontinued, because once it is, the preclinical symptoms return, often with greater intensity than before. This was discovered in another classic case.

Case History: Fran, age 13

Major Symptom: Violent temper tantrums

Diagnosis: Preclinical hypogeusia

Possible Cause: Corn and most corn products, high-fiber foods, especially bran; meat nurtured on copper-supplemented feed; peanuts; potatoes; soybeans and soybean products, including meat extenders

Dr. Carl C. Pfeiffer, one of the first nutrition scientists to link minerals to brain function, noted that Fran couldn't see things clearly and without distortion, forgot what was told her, had trouble learning, was chronically irritable, and was extremely antagonistic and uncooperative much of the time. But what particularly marked her disorder, Dr. Pfeiffer wrote, was "unprovoked temper tantrums involving ranting and raving [and] cruel swear words."

Before Fran's parents brought her to Dr. Pfeiffer in 1975, they had placed their daughter in the hands of psychiatrists, psychological counselors, and pediatricians with no results. But as soon as they told Dr. Pfeiffer the only time Fran was normal was after she had eaten fried oysters, he had the answers.

Oysters are rich in zinc, and they had temporarily wiped out the zinc deficiency that had triggered less intense symptoms of the zinc-deprivation disease, hypogeusia. Pointing out to her parents that Fran couldn't eat fried oysters three times a day for the rest of her life, he prescribed a zinc supplement in an amount appreciably higher than the RDA.

"The very next day they gave her the first dose of zinc," Dr. Pfeiffer wrote, "[and] she was positively improved. Within two weeks after she had started the zinc . . . the parents [were] enjoying the new Fran. [They were saying] 'She has a great sense of humor, is considerate and fun to be around.' She was always unusually alert and cooperative—and never had any tantrums."

But when, after three and a half months, her zinc supplements were discontinued, Fran "had a 'blowup'—a real temper tantrum . . . including ranting alone in her room," Dr. Pfeiffer wrote. "In a week . . . her behavior had deteriorated so much that [the parents] had to resume [zinc supplements].

"They gave her the first zinc capsule at 8:30 A.M.," Dr. Pfeiffer wrote. Then they watched and waited in a state of high anxiety to see if it would work again. By six that night their ordeal was over. Fran "was once again a changed person, and continued to be. 'There is no doubt whatsoever in our minds,' the parents told Dr. Pfeiffer, 'that zinc had saved her.' " Dr. Pfeiffer agreed.

Because Fran had continued on a diet which probably contained foods that caused the zinc deficiency, ODA supplementation had to be continued.

Our Eating Plan for Brighter Kids, ODA-supplemented for zinc, lets them enjoy all the anti-zinc foods that we've already listed in Fran's case history summary. It also helps protect against food cooked in copper pots. Although the right extremely small amount of copper is essential for the health of your kids (especially for the production in the body of the biochemical superoxide dimutose [SOD] which helps protect against certain carcinogenic agents), more than that amount is the deadly enemy of zinc.

The Complete Up-to-Date List of Anti-Vitamin, Anti-Mineral Foods—and How You Can Keep Them in Your Kids' Diet

The list starts on page 70. Certain amounts of these foods must be consumed before they have an effect on your kids' brains. These are the "trigger levels," and they differ from child to child. If your child's trigger levels are high, they may never be reached on an average diet.

Anti-Vitamin, Anti-Mineral Foods
That Could Brown Out Your Kids' Brains

Anti-Vitamin/Anti-Mineral Food	Vitamins/Minerals Attacked	Brain Brown-Out Symptoms
Almonds	Calcium	Anxiety, depression, irritability, insomnia, nervousness
Baking powder*	C	Hyperactivity, malaise, sluggishness, learning disability
Baking soda*	B_1, choline	Aggressive behavior, depression, fatigue, irritability, learning disability, memory loss, poor concentration
Beets	Calcium	See ALMONDS
Breakfast cereals	B_3	Hyperactivity, impaired sense perceptions, learning disability, irritability, memory loss, sluggishness
Brussels sprouts, raw	B_1, choline	See BAKING SODA
Cabbage, red, raw	B_1, choline	See BAKING SODA
Chocolate	B_{12}, inositol, calcium	Anxiety, depression, hyperactivity, insomnia, irritability, memory loss, mood swings, nervousness, poor concentration
Cocoa	See CHOCOLATE	See CHOCOLATE
Corn and most corn products (but not corn oil)	B_3, zinc	See BREAKFAST CEREALS symptoms; also extremely antagonistic behavior and violent temper tantrums
Coffee†	B_1, B_{12}, inositol	Aggressive behavior, depression, fatigue, irritability, learning disability, memory loss, mood swings, poor concentration
Egg whites, raw‡	Biotin	Fatigue, insomnia
Fiber foods, high (see page 85)	Calcium, magnesium, phosphorus, zinc, iron, copper	Anxiety, depression, diminished attention span, fatigue, hyperactivity, irritability, impaired sense perception, insomnia, lack of motivation, learning disability, memory loss, mood swings, nervousness, sluggishness

70

Food	Nutrient	Effects
Fish, raw	B_1, choline	See BAKING SODA
Grains, raw, unsprouted	B_3, inositol	Hyperactivity, impaired sense perception, insomnia, irritability, learning disability, memory loss, nervousness, sluggishness
Meat (from copper-supplemented feed)	Zinc	Violent temper tantrums, extremely antagonistic behavior, impaired sense perceptions, chronic irritability, learning disabilities, diminished attention span, fatigue
Peanuts	Zinc	See MEAT
Potatoes	Zinc	See MEAT
Rhubarb	Calcium	See ALMONDS
Saccharin	B_{12}, biotin	Fatigue, insomnia, memory loss, mood swings, poor concentration
Seeds	B_3, inositol	See GRAINS
Soybeans and soybean products (including meat extenders)	Zinc	See MEAT
Spinach	Calcium	See ALMONDS
Tea†	B_1, B_{12}, inositol	See COFFEE
Vegetable greens	B_3	See BREAKFAST CEREALS
Wine, red†	B_1, B_{12}, inositol	See COFFEE

* Baking soda is bicarbonate of soda. Baking powder also contains starch and either tartrate, calcium acid phosphate, or sodium aluminum sulfate plus calcium acid phosphate when it's called double-acting. Baking powder is used exclusively in baked goods; baking soda, in cooking vegetables as well.

† You probably wouldn't think of serving this beverage to your kids, but this is one more reason why you shouldn't.

‡ Products made from raw egg whites include meringues, Bavarian creams, mousses, chiffon pies, no-bake cakes and pies, and steak tartare.

NOTE: For anti-iron foods, see pages 82 and 83.

But even the highest trigger levels can be reached when one or more anti-vitamin or anti-mineral foods dominate a diet. Be careful of a diet of mostly high-fiber foods, for example (a list appears on page 85) that decimates six minerals; or a diet built around corn-based Tex-Mex foods that attacks vitamin B_3 and zinc. Be careful, too, of single meals especially high in anti-vitamin or anti-mineral foods. They could trigger flash preclinical symptoms of brain brown-out even in kids with high trigger levels. Such huge consumption may overwhelm the protection afforded by ODAs.

The effects of *moderate* amounts of anti-vitamin and anti-mineral foods in your kids' diet, though, can be offset by ODAs. The best possible children's diet supplies ODAs of *all* vitamins and minerals for two reasons. Medical nutrition science has just scratched the surface of knowledge about anti-vitamin, anti-mineral foods; and there may be foods your children are eating that, still unknown to us, together attack all vitamins and minerals. Vitamins and minerals are most effective when *all* are present in a child's brain (and body) in ODA quantities.

ODAs in the best possible diet come from three sources: from foods with the highest amounts of specific vitamins and minerals, from the proper mix of those foods to supply the highest levels of all vitamins and minerals, and from supplements to bring the levels up to ODA standards (which, unfortunately, in these days of foods that are vitamin-diminished by processing, can no longer be obtained from the foods themselves).

Our Eating Plan for Brighter Kids meshes these three sources for you into a protective diet against moderate use of anti-vitamin, anti-mineral foods. On it, your kids can enjoy all the nutritious foods on the anti-vitamin, anti-mineral foods list—and the foods likely to be added to it—without fear of brain brown-outs.

• CHAPTER •

7

THE AVERAGE AMERICAN DIET

Are Today's Fresh Foods as Bad as Junk Foods for Your Kids' Brains?

In the United States today, one out of three eighth-graders cannot read this sentence. "A tragedy," says the nation's leading expert on child care, Dr. Benjamin Spock.

Is this tragedy—the tragedy of kids who don't learn—rooted in the way kids eat? It's one root, many medical nutrition scientists believe, perhaps in our times the most important root.

From the identification of hyperactivity-inducing foods to the growing catalog of foods that can brown out kids' brains, blame has been laid on individual foods or groups of foods. But currently the indictment has shifted to the way kids eat—the total diet.

The average American diet for kids today is 80 percent junk food and 20 percent natural foods. Nutrition-minded parents, seeking a way to better the average, have cheered the appearance of rehabilitated junk foods—those with no or low sugar, salt, fat and additives; and those that are "all natural." They've also raised the percentage of *real* natural foods in their families' diets. But, sadly, most rehabilitated junk foods and most fresh foods are not as safe and sound as they seem.

Only a small number of rehabilitated junk foods meet the no-harm test; and most of our natural foods are in their own way as dangerously processed as junk foods. On the average American diet, no matter how you try to patch it, there is no way you can feed your kids to brightness, or to better health.

The evidence for that statement—highlights follow—is so compelling that you'll want to change your children's diet at once. It's the evidence that motivated us when we created our Eating Plan for Brighter Kids.

73

Aren't There Any Good Junk Foods?

Read the labels, and you'll find them perverse prescriptions for bringing on almost all the mental/emotional disorders scientists now associate with food:

Coloring, flavorings, preservatives, and other chemical additives that could afflict your kids with hyperactivity; sugar that could turn your kids into Jekyll-and-Hydes; caffeine (mainly in cola drinks and chocolate) that could lift your kids high then drop them to the bottom of the class; excess salt that, neurobiologists now claim, could overexcite your kids' brains; excess saturated fats that could slow them down.

Then add this data, which does not appear on the labels: Junk foods are processed food, and the very act of processing savagely reduces the vitamins and minerals necessary for the satisfactory functioning of your kids' brains.

It's because of these facts, labeled and unlabeled, that progressive medical professionals see junk foods as anti-learning foods. They have for some time also associated junk foods with degenerative diseases, like heart attack and diabetes, that frequently start, and often manifest themselves, in childhood. Assaulting both mind and body, junk foods, these scientists are convinced, are anti-kid foods.

So strong has the case against junk foods for kids grown in recent years that it has sparked a parents' rebellion, hitting the junk-food manufacturers where it hurts—at the check-out counter. Reform has followed; and now labels on containers of rehabilitated junk foods hard-sell NO or LOW or LESS junk-food ingredients, and ALL NATURAL ingredients.

But the reform is a giant step backward. Except for some items (there's a list on page 75), it fools people. Most junk foods remain junk foods.

Consider *no/low/less-sugar foods*. With some exceptions, they're laden with salt, additives, saturated fats, and substitute sweeteners that can be as harmful, or more harmful, than sugar. No-sugar soft drinks go cloudy without sugar, and something has to be added to give that crystal-clear sales appeal. That something is stannous chloride, and it can harm your kids' brains and nervous systems.

Consider *no/low/less-salt (sodium) foods*. Most of these are glutted with sugar or sugar substitutes and as gross a mix of additives and

The Best of the Rehabilitated Junk Foods

These products eliminate additives or limit them to one or just a few of the harmless ones (like BHT in shredded wheat), and contain no added sugar and little or no added salt. The canned foods on this list, although lacking the higher vitamin/mineral content of their natural counterparts, are sugar-free and salt-free or low in added salt, and are tasty additions to a well-balanced and fully supplemented diet. We include the best of the rehabilitated junk foods in our Eating Plan for Brighter Kids.

Baking powder, without aluminum (a mineral that could be harmful to your child's body and brain)

Canned pineapple in unsweetened pineapple juice

Canned salmon, sardines, and tuna, no salt added, packed in water

Canned whole tomatoes, tomato juice, tomato paste, tomato puree, no salt added

Dijon mustard, no salt or sugar added

Familia (Swiss Birchermuesli), the no-salt, no-sugar version of this breakfast food

Grain coffees (caffeine-free substitutes)*

Jams and jellies, unsweetened

Low-fat cheeses, low in salt

Pasta, salt-free and without additives—not new, but new in popularity in the USA

Peanut butter, unhydrogenated, unsalted, preferably freshly made

Rice crackers, Oriental, unsalted

Shredded wheat, including all new varieties

Soy sauce, sodium-reduced

Vegetable seasonings, low in salt

* For flavoring (as used in my recipes, grain coffees don't taste like coffee, so kids can't get hooked on the taste) and for adult enjoyment instead of real coffee.

saturated fats as you can find in any unreformed junk food. Low-sodium canned soups and most dry soup mixes are flagrant examples.

When sodium from sources other than salt (say, from *mono-sodium* glutamate [MSG]) is cut down in a food, more salt is usually added. So, there may not be a grain of MSG in some sausages anymore, but most are as salty as pickles. To make matters worse, they're also stuffed with saturated fats and additives.

Consider *no/low/less-fat foods*. These are crammed with almost all the junk that gives junk food its bad name—including saturated fats. Some health-food yogurt products—yogurt raisins, for example—are homogenized with highly saturated palm and coconut oils. (Oils are fats that are liquid at room temperature.)

Although there are some low-fat cheeses on the market, those sold as "skim" or "part-skim" aren't. The "skim" refers only to the milk employed at the start of the cheese-making process. Whole milk and cream must be added during the process to meet U.S. government standards for fat content, which is not low.

Consider *no/low/less-additives foods*. Some cut down on the number of additives, but one additive to a susceptible child could be as harmful as two dozen. Some truly include no additives during processing, but most of the foods have been treated chemically *before* they're processed—on the farm, in the orchards, at the ranch—and the additives are built-in. Your apple juice container may read PURE —NO ADDITIVES, but the apples come to the juice extractors already treated with pesticides, fungicides, coloring agents, and growth-control chemicals.

Consider *all-natural foods*. "Natural," by definition, is the opposite of "artificial." But since the Pure Food and Drug Administration has no jurisdiction over the word "natural," it would be unnatural for food processors not to define it as they choose. So one cheese is defined by its maker as "natural" that contains a coloring, excess salt, and a preservative—and that's typical of many "natural" foods.

At bottom, no contemporary processed food can truly be called natural because the very processing denaturalizes it—pillages it of the nutrients nature gave it. Canning destroys up to 80 percent of some minerals and up to 100 percent of some vitamins, according to Dr. Henry Schroeder, the nation's preeminent authority on the nutrient content of foods. Freezing is almost as devastating.

Milling so completely denudes grain of vitamins and minerals that the U.S. government has been forced to mandate that the mills "enrich" their flours with some of the nutrients they have stripped away. But, states Dr. Bernard Rimland, "there are well over twenty nutrients which lose 80 percent or so of their value in the milling process, and [the lost values of] only four of those twenty or so are replaced."

So, in a famous experiment conducted by the renowned pioneer medical nutrition scientist Dr. Roger J. Williams at the University of Texas, two-thirds of just-weaned rats on an "enriched" white-bread diet died in three months and the remaining one-third were abnormal. "If this 'food,'" comments Dr. Michael Colgan, "cannot support the life of a rat, a very tough, adaptable creature, then it certainly cannot support the life of a human child."

The New American Tragedy for Your Kids: Processed Fresh Food

The alternate to junk food is clearly natural food. But, sadly, the roughly 20 percent of our basic national diet that's not junk food is not really natural food either. It's a queer hybrid invented by modern agribusiness: processed fresh food.

The processing of fresh food begins in the soil. Treated with chemical growth-stimulants for decades, "our topsoil is becoming deficient," warns one of the nation's leading child-care specialists, Dr. Lendon Smith, former clinical professor of Pediatrics at the University of Oregon Medical School. "Even if we eat well, it is not a guarantee that we will get the minimum amount of minerals our bodies must have to function properly."

The minerals lacking in some of our nation's soil include iodine, iron, and zinc, whose deficiencies in kids' diets have been associated with preclinical and clinical mental/emotional problems and learning disabilities. Other minerals in short supply include calcium, copper, selenium, fluoride, and molybdenum. These, like the other three, are not only vital to a healthy body/brain for your kids, but also play important roles in the synthesis by plants of those vitamins, particularly of the B-complex, whose deficiencies can cripple the learning abilities of some children.

Grown nutrient-poor, some of our fruits and vegetables are further drained of nutrients by chemical control drugs that "promote uniform size, delay ripening so harvesting can take place at one time, intensify the color . . . and extend shelf life by two to three months," the Federal Environmental Protection Agency (EPA) reported in 1985. Millions of pounds of chemical control drugs are used yearly by growers of apples, Brussels sprouts, cantaloupes, sour cherries, Concord grapes, peaches, peanuts, prune plums, and tomatoes.

Penetrating skins and shells, these anti-nutrient chemicals bind to the interior of the produce, and cannot be removed by washing or cooking. Adding an estimated $31 million annual profit to the apple industry alone, chemical control drugs may also add suspected carcinogens to your kids' (and your) diet.

Other chemical processing agents intensify the assault on the nutrients in our plant food. Insecticides, pesticides, and fungicides play havoc with the vitamin/mineral content of edible skins, and some are goitrogens. Some skin colorings—those that brighten the hues of oranges, lemons, and limes, for example—are as savage in their attacks, and can cause hyperactivity in some kids when the rind is eaten, or sucked on, or used in cooking.

Skin colorings are also used to cosmeticize fruit and vegetables gathered before they're ripe. Unripe produce is an economic plus to agribusiness because these foods are harvested in the shortest time at the lowest cost, and they can endure on shelves longer before they rot. But unripe food has not had the time to manufacture its full quota of vitamins and other nutrients, and is not likely to do so after severance from the soil (bananas are the exception). The false ripe look of artificially colored produce is a cruel deception to parents who have come to regard fruit and vegetables as "good for their kids."

Another form of plant-food processing, refrigeration during shipping and storage to extend shelf life, takes a heavy toll on temperature-sensitive vitamins. Dr. Michael Colgan provides these examples: Lettuce, one day after it's picked, loses 50 percent of its vitamin C, and in three more days of subnormal temperatures loses 50 percent of the remaining vitamin, for a total loss of 75 percent. "Asparagus, broccoli, and green beans," he adds, "also lose . . . vitamin C in cold storage—50 percent *before* they reach your greengrocer" (emphasis ours).

Processing exacts its toll on our fresh animal food in many of the ways it does on our plant food. In two ways, though, the effects of the processing can be worse.

Synthetic hormones in feeds manufacture the most edible meat per production dollar, but the meat is supersaturated fatty, and abnormal in nutritive values. Antibiotics, processed into cattle, swine, turkey, and chicken, can induce allergic reactions, sometimes cerebral, in some kids, and may be goitrogenic. (Ironically, despite antibiotics, one out of three mass-produced chickens now can infect your kids [and you] with botulism, a bacterial food poisoning that can be fatal, unless you take the precooking precautions we prescribe on page 170.)

The shelf lives of some fresh animal and plant foods are now extended by streams of nuclear radiation. High-potency gamma rays from radioactive cobalt-60 and cesium-137, the stuff of nuclear fallouts, are blasted through fresh foods, destroying vitamins A, C, E, and especially vitamins of the B-complex, essential for the development and functioning of your children's brain and nervous systems. Athough food irradiation is regarded as "safe" by the food industry and the Food and Drug Administration, it is condemned as a major health hazard by many physicists, physicians, organizations concerned with public health, and some members of Congress.

To the degradation of fresh food by the food industry, add contamination from general industrial pollution. Mercury, cadmium, copper, aluminum, and lead in air, water, and soil infiltrate some of our fresh food at toxic levels, attacking children's bodies and brains directly, and by depriving them of vitamins and other essential minerals. It is no wonder that Dr. Bernard Rimland associates the metal poisoning of our foods with some of the most common mental diseases of today's children.

The fresh foods most of the nation's kids eat could be, at worst, as bad for them as junk foods; and, at best, suspect. ("It is impossible," states the Food and Drug Administration, "to establish with complete certainty the absolute harmlessness of any [added] chemical substance.") This puts you in a distressing situation. . . .

What CAN You Feed Your Kids?

You can feed your kids on the foods and supplements in our Eating Plan for Brighter Kids.

Processed fresh foods are here to stay, so realistically we use them —but in the best possible way: We select the most nutritious of them, and then protect your kids from their subnormal vitamin/ mineral content with ODA supplements. These also compensate for the vitamin/mineral losses in your kids' brains induced by some of the processing agents.

What our Plan does is enable you to feed your kids processed fresh foods—because they're the only fresh foods you can get— without harm to your kids' brains and bodies. It's the only do-able solution to today's denatured natural foods.

· CHAPTER ·
8

THE HIGH-CARBOHYDRATE DIET, THE WELL-BALANCED DIET

What's the Right Diet for Your Kids' Brains?

The leading alternates to the average American diet are the high-carbohydrate diet and the well-balanced diet.

The high-carbohydrate diet, currently enjoying a great vogue, is at the same time a low-protein, low-fat diet. The well-balanced diet, an invention of medical nutrition scientists at the U.S. Department of Agriculture (USDA) provides, as its name implies, an optimal balance—not too high, not too low—of carbohydrates, proteins, and fats.

Both of these well-respected diets may be harmful to your kids' brains. But one of them, the well-balanced diet, brought up to date and with the harmful factors removed, forms the base for the best possible diet not only for your children but for your whole family. It is the foundation diet for our Eating Plan for Brighter Kids.

Why the High-Carbohydrate Diet Can Harm Your Kids' Brains

Carbohydrates are one of the three classes of foods contributing energy (calories) to the human body/brain. They are found mainly in plant foods—vegetables, fruits, grains, legumes, and the products made from them. Indispensable to your kids' health and growth when consumed in the right amounts, they can savage the brain when they dominate the diet.

The RDA of carbohydrates for school kids is about 53 percent of the diet in terms of total calories; but some nutrition scientists consider 60 to 75 percent healthful. When the diet goes beyond 75 percent, it could be hazardous to your child. It is that kind of diet that we refer to as "the high-carbohydrate diet."

A high-carbohydrate diet can create iron deficiency, leading to kids' brain brown-outs:

Iron deficiency browns out a child's brain because the body lacks the right amount of iron to manufacture sufficient hemoglobin, the substance in red blood cells that transports oxygen to the brain. The brain then doesn't get enough oxygen, and this is what results:

Learning disabilities. Memory loss. Diminished attention span. Irritability. Sluggishness. Fatigue. Lack of motivation. All are preclinical symptoms of anemia. (Anemia is a disease of varied symptoms characterized by sickly red blood cells and a low red blood cell count.)

So devastating are the effects of brain oxygen shortage on a young child, even after it's corrected, that Dr. Ian Holzman, infant-care specialist at the Magee-Woman's Hospital, Pittsburgh, warns that early iron deficiency "could have significant [negative] implications in terms of learning and scholastic achievements" in later life.

No nutrition disorder is more widespread among young children than iron deficiency. We now know that anti-iron foods are one of its causes. This identification has come mainly as a result of the extensive and meticulous studies conducted by the medical nutrition scientists of the International Nutritional Anemia Consultive Group (INACG). A list of anti-iron foods, compiled from INACG data, appears opposite.

Anti-iron foods are harmful only on a high-carbohydrate diet, since they can successfully attack iron in plant foods (non-heme iron) but not in animal foods (heme iron). On a vegetarian diet, the presence of anti-iron foods means an iron-deficiency diet.

INACG warns, particularly, against a diet high in soybeans and soybean products, especially cereal-soy blends such as corn-soy-milk—a potent combination of anti-iron foods. The special danger, as INACG sees it, is that since soybeans are higher in proteins than other vegetables, they are widely used as inexpensive substitutes for animal protein to create a pure vegetarian diet with built-in iron-destructive capacity.

Foods That Can Cause Iron-Deficiency Brain Brown-Outs in Your Kids

•————————————•

These foods are harmless when animal foods are a regular part of your kids' diet, since anti-iron foods attack only iron present in plant foods (non-heme iron). Anti-iron foods on a pure vegetarian diet, which is low in iron to begin with, can be dangerous to your kids physically as well as mentally.

Anti-Iron Foods	Natural Anti-Iron Chemicals in the Foods
Bran	Phytates
Cereals	Phytates
Cheese	Phosphates
Corn	Phytates
Cowpeas (black-eyed peas)	Polyphenols
Eggs	Phosphates
Finger millet	Polyphenols
Horsebeans (broad beans)	Polyphenols
Legumes	Polyphenols
Milk, cow's*	Phosphates
Rice	Phytates
Sorghum	Polyphenols
Spinach	Polyphenols
Soybeans	Phytates and saponins
Tea†	Polyphenols
Wine, red†	Polyphenols

* This emphasizes the need of iron supplements for infants on formula, and for children who drink cow's milk.

† If you need another reason for eliminating these beverages from your kids' diet, here it is.

All anti-iron foods are harmless on a diet that supplies adequate amounts of meat, poultry, or fish. Meat, which is particularly high in heme iron, also increases the body's ability to use non-heme iron in the potatoes and other vegetables with which the meat is served. That's one reason meat—especially red meat, the highest in iron of all animal foods—is included in our Eating Plan for Brighter Kids.

Preclinical symptoms of anemia, and anemia itself, can also be induced on high-carbohydrate diets due to the virtual absence of vitamin B_{12} (cobalamin) and the extremely low levels of two other vitamins of the B-complex—vitamin B_6 (pyridoxine) and folic acid. All three vitamins are indispensable for the manufacture of hemoglobin.

These vitamins are supplied in the animal foods of our Eating Plan for Brighter Kids, and brought up to ODA levels with the *right* amount of supplements. (Taken in excess, iron may stimulate bacterial growth.) Our Plan is also rich in vitamin C (ascorbic acid), vital to the utilization of iron in the body/brain.

A high-carbohydrate diet can create deficiencies in six minerals, leading to kids' brain brown-outs:
A high-carbohydrate diet need not be high in fiber, but today it usually is. Fiber is what Grandma used to call "roughage." Fixed in the public's mind by media medical experts as "healthful," high-roughage diets can be rough on your kids.

Fiber is an indigestible carbohydrate (think of wood) that contributes no energy (calories) and no nutrients. It plays a necessary role in our digestive processes, helping to prevent constipation, and, by biochemical pathways still unknown, is purported to prevent a spectrum of diseases as far apart as tooth decay and diabetes.

The normal American diet for older school kids contains an estimated 6 to 10 grams (around a quarter of an ounce) of "dietary fiber" a day. (Dietary fiber describes all nonnutrient carbohydrates, as opposed to "crude fiber," which is applied to only two kinds.) High-fiber advocates recommend as much as 50 grams of dietary fiber daily—and that could be much too much for your kids.

At that level, fiber blocks the absorption of brain-vital minerals calcium, copper, iron, magnesium, phosphorus, and zinc. The result: Your kids can be afflicted by one, or any grouping, of the following preclinical symptoms.

Irritability. Nervousness. Insomnia. Mood swings. Anxiety.

High-Fiber Foods That May Harm Your Kids' Brain

• —————————————— •

High-fiber foods in moderation are unquestionably healthful, but prolonged consumption of above-optimal quantities can hurt your child mentally and physically. Not only does excess fiber impair the absorption of brain-vital minerals, but, attacked by intestinal bacteria, it produces noxious gases in the digestive track with possible consequent pain, vomiting, and nausea.

Beans (especially lima)
Berries (especially raspberries)
Bran cereals
Broccoli
Brussels sprouts
Coconut
Corn
Dried fruit (especially figs and raisins)
Fresh fruits (especially plums, pears, and apples *with* the skin)
Green beans
Legumes (especially peas)
Nuts (especially almonds)
Potatoes (especially baked with the skin)
Salad greens
Whole-wheat cereals

Depression. Memory loss. Diminished attention span. Impaired sense perceptions. Sluggishness. Fatigue. Lack of motivation. Learning disability.

It seems quite right then for the Food and Nutrition Board, National Academy of Sciences–National Research Council, to recommend that "marked increases in dietary fiber should be avoided."

Alice White, the noted children's nutritionist, adds another reason for curbing fiber consumption:

"High-fiber foods tend to be low in calories, and since your children have small stomachs, emphasis on these foods might not provide your child with adequate calories"—and without adequate calories, the supply of all nutrients is inadequate.

"Parents should add fiber to meals in moderation," cautions Boston Children's Hospital, the nation's largest pediatric medical center. Our Eating Plan for Brighter Kids limits the amount of high-fiber foods to moderate, healthful levels.

The high-carbohydrate diet can create protein and fat deficiencies, leading to kids' brain brown-outs.

The protein RDA for school kids is 8 percent of the diet in terms of total calories. Below the RDA, kids are liable to show symptoms of the protein-deprivation disease kwashiorkor, now afflicting millions of kids on pure vegetable diets in Ghana, Southeast Asia, Central America, and South America. Kwashiorkor in the language of the Gold Coast (now Ghana), where it was first discovered by the pioneer British medical nutrition scientist Dr. Cicely D. Williams, means "the disease that causes kids to lose touch with reality."

There's no known kwashiorkor in the United States. But when kids' protein consumption drops to between 8 and 12 percent of the diet—known as the protein gap—preclinical symptoms of kwashiorkor can develop. On a high-carbohydrate diet, particularly a pure vegetarian diet, your kids' protein consumption could drop into the protein gap. When that happens, your kids could experience some or all of these symptoms:

Impaired sense perceptions. Slow-down of brain activity that could lead to mental retardation. Memory loss. Emotional instability. Mood swings. Confusion. Depression. Loss of interest in people and surroundings. Feelings of worthlessness. Stress. Anxiety. Sleeplessness. Nail biting. Chronic fatigue. Dizziness.

The protein gap can also be harmful in another way. Proteins in nature are packaged with vitamins and minerals necessary for the health of your kids' brains. When your kids' brains are getting subhealthful quantities of proteins, they're also getting subhealthful quantities of those nutrients.

Medical nutrition scientists have reported such high vitamin/mineral deficiencies on a protein-gap diet (particularly of vitamins A and folic acid, and minerals iron, zinc, manganese, magnesium, and copper) that Dr. Alan Jackson terms the proteins on such a diet "empty proteins"—a counterpart of empty calories. Dr. Jackson is the director of the Tropical Metabolism Research Unit, University of West Indies, Jamaica.

The vitamin/mineral deficiencies induced by the protein gap on a high-carbohydrate diet are intensified by a level of fat so low that it may induce "fat starvation" in some children. In this condition, there is not enough fat in the child's bloodstream to transport sufficient fat-soluble vitamins (A, D, E and K) to sites in the brain where they are vitally needed.

Overall, a high-carbohydrate diet, by sharply reducing proteins and fats, can bring about preclinical symptoms in your kids of many vitamin/mineral–deprivation diseases.

Our Eating Plan for Brighter Kids, accordingly, is not a high-carbohydrate diet. It's a diet with balanced amounts of carbohydrates, proteins, and fats—but it's not *the* "well-balanced diet" invented by the USDA.

Why the USDA's Well-Balanced Diet Can Harm Your Kids

This is the diet many nonnutrition doctors tell you to put your kids on, and go on yourself, to solve all nutritional ills.

It's based on tables compiled by the USDA of the nutrient contents, in numbers, of virtually every American food. By reference to these numbers, USDA nutritionists have calculated how many servings of selections from each of the four Food Groups provide 100 percent of the RDAs for children and adults. (The Food Groups are vegetables/fruits, bread/cereals, milk/cheese, meat/poultry/fish/beans.) The USDA provides lists of foods in each Group, and a formula for creating daily menus based on the right number of servings from each group.

Brilliantly conceived, the well-balanced diet became the one reliable guidepost in the labyrinth of conflicting diet claims.

Then, in 1973, Dr. Michael Colgan made a startling discovery: In his clinic, three-quarters of the patients on the well-balanced diet

showed signs of malnutriton. Shocked, Dr. Colgan and his col-
leagues "then began to measure the vitamin and mineral content of
. . . the foods [the patients] actually ate. We were amazed to find,"
he reported, "that even fresh raw fruits did not contain anything
like the amounts of nutrients given in the nutrient tables."

Dr. Colgan's team laboratory-analyzed supermarket oranges. According to the tables, the analyses should have revealed a vitamin-
C content of 90 milligrams per orange. "One batch of oranges
looked, smelled, and tasted perfectly usual," Dr. Colgan wrote.
"Their vitamin C content was zero." Not all batches of oranges
showed this stunning diminution of vitamin C, but the vitamin-C
content of each batch was markedly subpar.

Further laboratory tests on such common foods as carrots, cheddar cheese, eggs, liver, tomatoes, wheat germ, and stone-ground
whole-wheat flour revealed similar large deviations from values in
nutrient tables.

The enormous gap between nutrient-table figures and the real
ones, in Dr. Colgan's opinion, makes nonsense of nutrient tables—
and of the common advice proffered by doctors and nutritionists
that the well-balanced diet provides ample nutrition. "Diets are deficient," he concludes, "when they are planned from tables of nutrient contents of foods."

The prime cause of the vast discrepancies between the tabular
values of nutrients in foods and the real values, is that most of the
tabular values were determined before the full impact of mass food
processing, even of fresh foods, had taken its toll.

But even if the nation's foods were still as nutritious as they once
were, the well-balanced diet cannot, because of flaws in the USDA's
formula for creating daily menus, always produce RDAs of all nutrients.

On one heavily medically endorsed version of this diet, Drs.
Michelle Fisher and Paul LaChance of Rutgers University found
significant shortfalls in vitamins B_1, B_6, and B_{12}, and in minerals zinc,
iron, magnesium, and calcium. Even the USDA concedes that, with
its formula for utilizing the Food Groups, it is impossible to design
well-balanced daily menus that meet the minimal needs of women
and children for vitamins B_6 and folic acid, and for the minerals iron
and zinc.

But the major drawback is this: At best, the well-balanced diet
can only contribute RDAs, not the ODAs necessary to ward off

preclinical disorders that disrupt your kids' mental, emotional, and behavioral well-being. When this diet supplies even less than RDAs the danger to your kids is heightened.

The Right Diet for Your Kids' Brains

Yet the basic idea of the well-balanced diet is sound, and recently nutrition scientists have discovered how to eliminate the defects in the USDA version. By arranging foods into more than four Food Groups, and applying a new formula, they can create menus with maximum real, not tabular, values. But these values still don't meet ODA levels, and full vitamin/mineral supplementation is necessary to do so.

With these improvements, the USDA well-balanced diet ceases to be a threat to kids, and becomes a healthful diet that can increase their learning ability and brightness.

For the children on such a diet, Dr. Colgan observed striking improvements in their emotions, behavior, speech articulation, reading skills, and overall classroom performance. "What we did not expect," he writes, "were improvements in intelligence quotients. But we found improvements of between *5 and 35 I.Q. points* with an average improvement of 17.9 points" (emphasis his).

The Nutrition/ Brightness Revolution in Brain Research

9

THE BIRTH OF YOUR CHILD'S BRAIN

Feeding Yourself Right and Your Kids Bright During Pregnancy

In the last ten years or so, a new breed of scientists, the neurobiologists, have discovered more about how your child's brain grows in your womb than humankind had learned in all its previous long years on earth.

In practical terms, this revolutionary new knowledge provides you for the first time with a guide to the foods of pregnancy that help you give birth not only to a healthy child but to a bright child. It keys you to:

- the best foods for growing your child's brain cells (billions of them) and the amazing communications network that connects them

- the best foods for building a special group of brain cells that increase your unborn child's brain power (the glial-cell complex; Albert Einstein had a larger glial-cell complex than most people)

- the best foods for providing your unborn child's brain cells with the energy to grow on (they have to supply just the *one* nutrient your kid's brain will accept)

- the best food supplements, because without them all the other "bests" would be second bests

- and the worst foods that, if relied on mainly during pregnancy, could harm your baby's brain.

Remember: During pregnancy, what *you* eat is what your unborn child's brain grows on. When you eat bright for your child, you eat right for yourself—including a surprising plus: You may not have to gain all that weight most doctors say you have to (see pages 105–7).

The Best Foods for Growing Your Unborn Child's Brain Cells and the Brain's Communication Network

The brain is protein territory.

The basic brain cell (the neuron) is mainly protein. The part of the brain cell that carries messages like a telephone wire (the axon) is a protein. So are the parts that send messages to other cells (the axon terminals) and receive messages from other cells (the dendrites). The remarkable biochemicals that activate brain messages (the neurotransmitters) are proteins. The substance in the brain that manages the growth of this total communications network, the Nerve Growth Factor, NGF, is a protein.

Should you go on a high-protein diet during pregnancy?
You should not.

For decades doctors prescribed high-protein pregnancy diets (they've only discontinued the practice in the last several years), and none of the kids were any brighter for it. (The doctors weren't trying for brighter kids; they were trying to prevent a common pregnancy disorder, toxemia. They didn't.)

Actually, the growing brain can handle just so much protein, and blocks out the rest. What your kid's brain needs is not massive doses of protein, but the right amounts of the right proteins.

The right amounts are easily obtained from animal food—meat, fish, poultry, cheese, milk, and plain yogurt—from about a quarter pound a day for a 100-pound woman to about a half pound for a 165-pound woman (weights are prepregnancy). These animal foods also supply the right proteins.

They're called "complete proteins" because they contain in the right proportions the complete roster of the amino acids your kid's growing body and brain need from foods. These are the "essential amino acids," and you can find out fast how important they are to your kid's brain from the chart on page 96.

Are vegetable proteins as good for your unborn child as animal proteins?
Most plant foods do not contain all the amino acids. Some plant foods contain some of them; some contain others. In the plant foods that do contain all the amino acids, the proportions are wrong for human needs. The only way to obtain complete proteins for your unborn child from plant foods is to combine specific selections from the vegetable kingdom that together provide all the essential amino acids in the right proportions.

Here is a sampling of such combinations. They're called *complementary proteins:*

Rice and sesame seeds	Beans and corn bread
Rice and tofu	Beans and tortillas
Rice and beans	Garbanzo beans and tahini
Rice and lentils	(sesame-seed paste)
Beans and peas	Soybeans (roasted),
Beans and whole-wheat	sunflower
bread	seeds, and peanuts
Beans and cracked wheat	Lentils and barley
Beans and cornmeal	Split peas and corn bread

Whether it's prudent on a pregnancy diet to replace complete animal proteins with complementary vegetable proteins is a matter of controversy.

In favor are the nutritionists who point out that in some animal protein–impoverished countries, diets of complementary proteins —such as rice and beans, or corn-based tortillas and beans—provide the amino acids essential to unborn children. Patricia Houseman, formerly staff nutritionist at the Center for Science in the Public Interest, Washington, D.C., writes that "the record shows that vegetable protein *can* meet the protein needs of . . . pregnant and nursing women" (emphasis ours).

But the opponents of a vegetarian diet point out that a high-carbohydrate diet may prevent amino acids from reaching the unborn child's brain. This diet is also likely to be low in the vitamin folic acid and the minerals calcium, iron, and zinc, all necessary for the construction of brain proteins from amino acids.

Essential Amino Acids: The Brain Brighteners
• ——————————————— •

For any of the amino acids to be effective, all must be present in the body/brain in optimal amounts. Those amounts of essential amino acids are supplied by the animal and vegetable foods of our Eating Plan for Brighter Kids. Because of the chance of overdosage from amino acid supplements with consequent harm to kids' brains, these supplements should not be given to kids, and should not be taken by you during pregnancy and breastfeeding. The essential amino acids listed here are essential for children; not all are essential for adults.

Arginine releases the growth hormone (GH) which is crucial to brain and body growth.

Cystine/Cysteine helps protect against mental disorders.

Glutamine stimulates mental activity, diminishes confusion, improves memory and learning ability.

Glycine produces a calming effect in stress situations.

Histidine promotes brain growth.

Isoleucine helps prevent mental retardation.

Leucine improves mental activity and fights mental disorders.

Lysine helps the brain utilize calcium, a mineral vital to neuronal functioning.

Methionine combats stress and fatigue, and helps ward off mental disorders.

Phenylalanine strengthens neurotransmitter signals. With tyrosine, it promotes alertness, ambition, and positive feelings— including feelings of joy.

Taurine improves memory.

Threonine contributes to normal brain functioning.

Tryptophan stabilizes emotions, reverses depression, suppresses irrational anger, and normalizes sleep patterns.

Tyrosine boosts intelligence, helps control anxiety and depression, provides a lift from fatigue. (See *Phenylalanine.*)

Valine promotes mental vigor, dissipates negative emotions.

In addition, a pure vegetarian diet contains virtually zero vitamin B_{12}, leading to brain-damaging preclinical and clinical anemia. And recently discovered is the association of mental disorders with severe vitamin-A deficiency in the diets of unborn children in animal protein–impoverished countries.

Boston Children's Hospital, basing its conclusion on physical health hazards alone, asserts that "vegan diets which omit all sources of animal protein . . . are not suitable and, in fact, are dangerous for growing children."

Three compromise diets, devoid of animal flesh but containing some animal food, hold out the promise of complete protein without the drawbacks of a pure vegetarian diet. They are:

The lacto-ovo-vegetarian diet. "Lacto" means milk and cheese; "ovo" means eggs; and vegetarian means vegetables, fruits, grains, legumes plus nuts. *The lacto-vegetarian diet* excludes eggs, and features milk and cheese with any of the following: potatoes, beans, rice, peanuts, or wheat. *The ovo-vegetarian diet* substitutes eggs for milk and cheese. All these diets include products made from the basic ingredients.

These diets are basically sound, but since the match of plant foods with animal foods must be made with extreme care to provide a complete protein, they are not recommended during pregnancy unless under doctor/nutritionist supervision.

Should you get the essential amino acids your unborn child needs from amino acid supplements?

No. Your unborn child's brain can shut out excess amino acids from protein *foods*, but it cannot shut out excess amino acids from *supplements*. Excess quantities of amino acids may induce overexcitement in the growing brain, leading at birth to a child prone to mental disorders as serious as hyperactivity, and intense anxiety leading to panic.

That's one reason some nutrition scientists recommend banning from your kitchen the sweetener aspartame, even though it's FDA approved. It's actually an amino acid supplement composed of two amino acids, phenylalanine and aspartic acid. Boston Children's Hospital reports that "consumer advocacy groups . . . contend that the body cannot metabolize . . . high concentrations of amino acids efficiently, and that health problems, even brain damage . . . may result if growing children use too much aspartame."

Amino acids are best derived from the protein in your diet. But be careful:

- Don't binge on a high-carbohydrate meal. The carbohydrates stimulate the flow of insulin, and that expels most of the amino acids from your bloodstream before they can reach your unborn child's brain.

- Stay away from the sprouts of navy, pinto, and kidney beans. They interfere with the body's metabolic processes that extract the amino acids from protein food. Most sprouts are healthful, but these can deprive your unborn child's brain of essential amino acids.

How can you benefit during pregnancy from the right amounts of the right proteins?

These help you to a successful pregnancy in the following ways: by providing normal growth of your breasts, blood volume, and

---

Guidelines to Protein Sources for Your Pregnancy Diet

• ———————————————————— •

These are the guidelines we followed in creating our Eating Program for Brighter Kids.

The Best Protein Foods: Animal foods—meat, fish, poultry, eggs, cheese, milk, and plain yogurt; and complementary vegetable foods (see list on page 95). These foods supply the essential amino acids for your unborn child's growing brain.

The Worst Protein Foods: Vegetable foods when they're not complemented—vegetables, fruits, grains, and legumes. These foods lack some of the essential amino acids on which your child's brain will grow. However, foods from the vegetable kingdom are indispensable on a well-balanced pregnancy diet to provide energy for the growth of your child's brain.

uterus; building stronger enzyme, hormone, hemoglobin, and immune systems; and by producing optimal quantities of amniotic fluid, the colorless liquid that protects your baby during gestation.

The Best Foods for Increasing Your Unborn Child's Brain Power

Associated with I.Q., the glial-cell complex of the brain strengthens your unborn child's brain power in several ways.

The complex is a storehouse of nutrients—of amino acids, vitamins, and minerals for building neurons and the brain's communications network; and of glucose to power brain growth and activity. It helps form a superthick "blood-brain" barrier, that keeps out many substances in the blood that could dim the developing brain. It provides the insulation for the brain's wiring system that strengthens the electrical impulses that "fire" the brain's activity.

When the glial-cell complex is not constructed properly, your child could be born with an impaired brain. But constructed properly, your child's brain could reach its maximum brightness.

The glial-cell complex is constructed mostly of fats and cholesterol.

Should you go on a high-fat, high-cholesterol diet during pregnancy?

Yes, according to Dr. Ralph Minear, the nation's leading authority on eating programs for feeding kids' brains. With the growth needs of the glial-cell complex in mind, he sets the fat-consumption figure during pregnancy at 50 percent of the diet in terms of total calories.

He also holds that "cholesterol [is] obviously . . . absolutely essential . . . to the child's . . . proper brain development [and] mental well-being." Consumption of cholesterol after conception, he asserts, should not be curbed.

The position of Dr. Minear, who is a pediatrician at Harvard Medical School, is sharply at variance with that of most of the nation's doctors who have established the low-fat, low-cholesterol diet as a principle of good health. That diet, which is purported to fight atherosclerosis (which can lead to heart attack) and other degenerative diseases including diabetes and cancer, contains sparse amounts of cholesterol and 20 percent less fat than permitted by Dr. Minear.

How, then, can the high-fat/cholesterol recommendation of Dr. Minear be reconciled with the high-fat/cholesterol condemnation of virtually the rest of the medical profession?

Dr. Minear answers, "There is a strong line of [medical] opinion that says giving a child significant amounts of cholesterol will help [the child's] body process it better later—and will . . . protect [the child] in . . . adult years against atherosclerosis." Other nutrition scientists believe that a fully vitamin/mineral–supplemented diet during pregnancy protects mother and child from faulty fat/cholesterol metabolism that may lead to atherosclerosis.

"As for myself," Dr. Minear, who recommends full supplementation, states, "I'm convinced that the need of [the child's] growing brain for fats and cholesterol . . . far outweighs any . . . fears about hardening of the arteries [atherosclerosis]." A low-fat/cholesterol diet may be beneficial to adults and older children, Dr. Minear concludes, but a high-fat/cholesterol diet is beneficial to unborn and younger children.

What are the best fats for your unborn child's growing brain?

There are three kinds of fats. *Saturated fats,* which are found in meat and poultry, are implicated in the onset of atherosclerosis. *Polyunsaturated fats,* which are vegetable fats (except palm and coconut oils, which are saturated fats) have been recommended as a safe replacement for saturated fats; but recent evidence indicates that under certain circumstances they can change in the body and brain to destructive substances. The trend now is to opt for *monounsaturated fats*—some vegetable fats—such as olive oil and peanut oil —that seem to have no harmful effects.

However, the fats your child's growing brain needs must contain the essential fatty acids (EFAs)—linoleic, linolenic, and arachidonic —and all these fats are polyunsaturated. Nutrition scientists point out that they cannot be transformed to harmful substances in the body and brain when the diet is fully supplemented. The best sources of polyunsaturated fats are virgin vegetable oils (first-pressed) and fish.

Cholesterol is, contrary to popular belief, not a fat, but a waxy alcohol. It's found in animal foods. There's no cholesterol in the vegetable kingdom. That's another reason a pure vegetarian diet during pregnancy is dangerous to your child's brain.

How can you benefit during pregnancy from the right amount of the right fats?

Fats are necessary for the structural changes in your body to prepare for the birth and nursing of your child, particularly the enlargement of the uterus and breasts. Cutting down on fats during pregnancy, from the physiological viewpoint alone, can be harmful to both you and your child. But don't regard this as a license to

Guidelines to Fat and Cholesterol Sources for Your Pregnancy Diet

• ———————————— •

These are the guidelines we followed in creating our Eating Program for Brighter Kids.

The Best Fat Foods: Vegetable oils that contain high amounts of essential fatty acids, such as almond, corn, safflower, sesame (not the Oriental variety), soybean, sunflower and walnut oils. Fish and other marine animals. Butter, sweet (no salt), natural or colored only with beta-carotene, which is beneficial.

The Worst Fat Foods: Animal fats (except fish fats), hydrogenated fats.

The Best Cholesterol Foods: Whole milk, eggs, dairy products, meat (especially organ meats like liver), fish and other marine animals.

The Worst Cholesterol Foods: Vegetables, grains, legumes, skim milk, nonfat milk, and products made from these. These are nutritious foods; and although whole milk is preferred to skim milk during pregnancy, all the others are part of our balanced pregnancy menus. They are not preferred as foods to be eaten exclusively during pregnancy.

gorge on fatty foods. Follow the moderate guidelines of our Eating Plan for Brighter Kids.

The Best Foods for Providing Your Unborn Child's Brain with the Energy to Grow On

Without glucose, the brain is powerless, literally without power. But when glucose is bonded with another substance in the brain, ATP, energy is generated that builds the brain and makes it run. Close down the flow of glucose, and the brain dims down and eventually dies.

Glucose is a member of a class of foods called saccharides that includes sugars and starches. Sucrose, also a saccharide, breaks down in the body to fructose and glucose.

Is sucrose a good source of glucose, the brain's energy food?
Not commercial sucrose—the pure, white crystalline sugar that has been stripped of every vitamin and mineral needed for its metabolism by the body. *That* sucrose is abnormally metabolized, producing chemicals that could be harmful to your unborn child's (and your) body/brain.

But in nature, sucrose—in unprocessed fresh fruits, berries, and vegetables—is always packaged with the vitamins and minerals needed to be utilized normally by the body. The highest sucrose-content food of all, sugar cane, is brimful of metabolism-necessary vitamins and minerals; and it's been a tasty, nutritious staple of tropical peoples for millennia. (Perhaps it's time to revive it in our supermarkets as the "new" health-food sweet.)

Can you get your supply of glucose during pregnancy from glucose tablets?
No. Because the pure, white crystalline glucose in these tablets is empty calories, stripped of all the vitamins and minerals essential to its metabolism. Glucose tablets can be as harmful to your unborn child's brain as pure sucrose.

All naturally occurring saccharides are converted in the body to glucose, so look for your best sources of glucose in foods which supply the most glucose from their saccharides. You'll find a list of

The Best Sources of Glucose—the Nutrient That Powers Your Unborn Child's Brain Growth and Function

• ————————————— •

Although most of the foods on this list do not contain glucose as such, they metabolize to glucose in the body. The "glucose value" represents the amount of glucose supplied by a food compared to that supplied by pure glucose, which has a glucose value of 100. Do not settle on just one of these foods for its high glucose value, but eat a variety of them to obtain a maximum mix of other nutrients.

Food	Type of Saccharide	Glucose Value
Fruits	Glucose, fructose, sucrose	80 to 95
Berries	Glucose, fructose, sucrose	80 to 95
Grains	Starch	65 to 90
Vegetables	Starch, sucrose	60 to 90
Potatoes	Starch	80
Mushrooms	Starch	40 to 50
Milk	Lactose	30 to 50
Oysters	Glycogen	20 to 25
Liver	Glycogen	10

those foods on this page. It's based on the studies of Dr. Arne Dahlqvist, professor and chairman of Nutrition, the University of Lund, Sweden.

How can you benefit during pregnancy from high glucose–value foods?
These power-packed foods provide the energy for the structural and hormonal changes necessary for a successful pregnancy. They also help prevent one of the common complaints of pregnant women—"that worn-out feeling."

Guidelines to Glucose Sources for Your Pregnancy Diet

• ————————————— •

These are the guidelines we followed in creating our Eating Program for Brighter Kids.

The Best Glucose Foods: See the table on page 103.

The Worst Glucose Foods: Pure white, crystalline sucrose, glucose, and other sugars, and their products. All animal foods except oysters, milk, animal livers. But animal foods are otherwise essential and are part of our balanced pregnancy menus.

The Best Vitamin Supplements for Getting the Most from the Best Foods During Pregnancy

The nutrients with which you feed your unborn child bright and yourself right during pregnancy—complete proteins, essential amino and fatty acids, cholesterol and high-glucose foods—cannot be utilized fully without all vitamins and minerals present in your body at full strength. Vitamins and minerals are "co-factors" that enter into the biochemical processes building your unborn child's body/brain, and prepare your body for childbirth.

That deficiencies in vitamins and minerals during pregnancy can adversely affect your child's mental health has been well-established. Dr. Michael Colgan, as a result of a survey conducted in 1983, reported that "the diets of teen-age girls are seriously deficient in calcium, iron, magnesium, and vitamin B_6. . . . For the pregnant among these girls, their babies risk . . . mental retardation."

On the other hand, complete supplementation during pregnancy could help you give birth to a potentially bright child. Dr. Josep Brožek of the Psychology Department, Lehigh University, Pennsylvania, reviewing the scientific literature over the last fifteen years on the nutrition/brightness link, concludes that prenatal supplementation improves a child's mental performance later in life, particularly in the areas of memory, language, and perception.

When should you start to take vitamin/mineral supplements, and in what amounts?

Progressive nutrition scientists hold that supplementation should begin prior to conception to compensate for ODA–vitamin/mineral deficiencies suffered by most women on typical American diets. Bringing vitamin/minerals in the body up to ODA levels, these scientists agree, helps you enter pregnancy in optimal health to produce a bright and healthy child.

During pregnancy, however, some doctors recommend RDA supplements lest higher amounts have an adverse effect on the unborn child's growing brain. Dr. Bernard Rimland dissents. "There is no evidence for this," he writes, "except that truly *massive* amounts of vitamin A could produce defects in a small number of sensitive individuals" (emphasis his).

He reports one study in which pregnant women were provided with 10,000 milligrams of vitamin C a day instead of the pregnancy RDA of 60 milligrams. "The children were unusually bright and healthy, and there never was a retarded one." The same study, and others, also revealed an advantage to the pregnant women from high vitamin-C dosage: "The duration of labor was cut in half."

Dr. Rimland also holds that the much-publicized claim that "megadoses of vitamin B_6 taken by pregnant women will lead to vitamin-B_6 dependency in the offspring is not proven and probably incorrect." For pregnant women, he concludes, "I would certainly opt for Optimal Dietary Allowance [ODA] levels."

How can you benefit from taking all the right vitamins and minerals in the right amounts during pregnancy?

Aside from maintenance of your wellness, and the natural high that comes from good nutrition, you can benefit from it in a surprisingly pleasant way: It can help keep your weight down. Here are the facts:

During pregnancy a woman's vitamin and mineral needs increase (even pregnancy RDAs are higher than nonpregnancy RDAs). To meet these needs, pregnant women eat more; and the increased calorie consumption accounts for most of the weight gain.

On the average pregnancy diet of the early 1950s, built mainly on nonprocessed foods naturally rich in vitamins and minerals, the increase in calories necessary to supply the vitamin/mineral needs of pregnancy resulted in weight gains of only 10 to 15 pounds.

But as the food processing industry progressively cut the vitamin/mineral content of American food, it became necessary for women to eat more *and more* to obtain their pregnancy vitamin/mineral ODAs. Weight gains during pregnancy mounted. By the early 1960s, the medically approved weight gain had soared to 20 pounds; by the early 1970s to 24 to 27 pounds; and currently it's at an all-time high of 30 pounds.

Guidelines for Vitamin/Mineral Supplements to Your Pregnancy Diet

• ——————————————— •

These are the guidelines we followed in creating our Eating Program for Brighter Kids.

The Best Vitamin/Mineral Supplements: See Chapter 16 for suggested ODA formulations. Remember, your individual nutritional needs probably are different from any other woman's. Follow the recommendations of a doctor trained and experienced in nutrition.

The Worst Vitamin/Mineral Supplements: Those differing in ingredients or values from those recommended by your nutrition-trained and -experienced doctor. Do not rely on just some vitamins and minerals; vitamins and minerals are most effective when *all* are present in the right amounts.

While most nonpregnant American women consume 1,200 to 1,600 calories a day, many doctors recommend 2,600 to 2,800 calories for pregnant women—which can result in prodigious weight gains (one slim woman added 68 pounds). Even the now "normal" weight gain of 30 pounds is a burden to many women, who find the excess poundage put on easily during pregnancy is hard to take off afterward.

A diet that leads to prolonged obesity is a health hazard. It should be avoided at any time. Studies by Dr. John Dobbing of the Manchester Medical School in England reveal it may be avoided in pregnancy with "increased dietary efficiency"—getting the most nutritive value out of just-right amounts of foods. This may be accomplished by a sound balanced diet, fully supplemented. In this way, a woman could consume her pregnancy ODAs, and be "relieved of the need to eat more during pregnancy" to obtain them. Whether "increased dietary efficiency" can restore average pregnancy weight gains to the 10-to-15 pound level of the 1950s is still to be determined. But the new concept holds out hope for today's weight-conscious mothers-to-be.

A word of caution: Before you go on a fully supplemented diet during pregnancy—and especially if you desire to control your weight—it is mandatory to consult a pediatrician who is trained and experienced in nutrition.

· CHAPTER ·

10

THE SECOND BIRTH OF YOUR CHILD'S BRAIN

The Bright Foods of Infancy and Early Childhood

Most children are born with about 10 billion basic brain cells (neurons). But after birth not a single neuron will ever be born again. If for any reason, nutritional or otherwise, your child is born with less than the full quota of neurons, there's no cause to despair. Nature has built a unique fail-safe mechanism. In essence, your child's brain is born for a second time—after birth.

This is one of the most dazzling discoveries of today's neurobiologists. As described by Dr. Jean-Pierre Changeux, professor of Neurobiology at the College de France, Paris, and a leader in the recent triumphs of brain research concerning children, the second birth involves the natural construction of a "new" brain using the billions of neurons with which your child was born.

This involves an intricate growth process, according to Dr. Changeux, in which three basic elements of the brain proliferate in immense numbers to form "pathways in the brain"—communication circuits with which your child talks, feels, thinks, acts. These "pathways"—in an almost infinite variety—transform the virtually unorganized brain at birth into the amazing machine with which your child will perceive the world and react to it.

The three basic elements that multiply enormously after birth are the glial-cell complex, the neurotransmitters, and the dendrites. For glial-cell expansion your child's brain needs fats and cholesterol; for neurotransmitters and dendrites, proteins; for the energy of growth, glucose. And for the co-factors that activate all these nutrients, your child needs the full quota of vitamins and minerals. The nutritional demands of your child's brain after birth—and for

108

three to five years thereafter as the new brain grows faster than it ever will again—are fundamentally the same as they were during pregnancy, only intensified.

How is your infant and your young child to be fed during this period? Nature has developed the perfect food—mother's milk. But if you plan to discontinue breastfeeding after at most six months, as most American mothers do, don't worry—our Eating Plan for Brighter Kids provides a basic nutritional equivalent of mother's milk for the full span of the second birth of your child's brain.

Breastfeeding: The Best Way to Feed Your Infant to Brightness

The current position of the medical profession, as reflected by Dr. William C. McClean, Jr., clinical associate professor of Pediatrics at Ohio State University, is: "Human milk is a *complete* food able to meet the nutritional requirements of the newborn and older infant. . . . *There is no doubt that breastfeeding is preferred for the infant*" (emphasis ours).

Mother's milk has been perfectly bioengineered by nature to satisfy all the nutritional needs of the second birth of your child's brain.

It contains all the essential amino acids in the right proportions. (The wrong proportions can stunt brain growth, distort neurotransmitter balance, and lead to brain disorders.) The quality of a protein is measured by how closely the proportions of its amino acids resemble proportions of amino acids in the human body. This comparison is called the biological value, and is rated on the basis of 0 to 100. Mother's milk has a biological value of 100. (Only egg white at 94 comes close.)

Mother's milk contributes a rich supply of fats to support the rapid growth of the glial-cell complex, which nurtures and protects the explosively expanding pathways in the brain. The fats are mainly unsaturated, the kind not associated with heart attack.

But these fats are vulnerable to attacks of "oxidants," vicious chemical fragments in the body/brain that can degenerate polyunsaturated fats into brain poisons. Mother's milk destroys these oxidants with an anti-oxidant nutrient team that includes vitamins A, E, C, B_1, and B_5; the minerals selenium, copper, and manganese; and the amino acids cystine and methionine.

Disturbing to the vast majority of doctors who now associate cholesterol with atherosclerosis and other degenerative diseases is the rich supply of cholesterol in mother's milk—a supply necessary to nurture the glial-cell complex. But cholesterol has been in mother's milk since the human race began without inducing those diseases. It's possible that mother's milk in well-nourished mothers contains a protective battery of vitamins and minerals that prevents faulty metabolism leading to the arterial deposits of cholesterol that are one of the causes of atherosclerosis.

Boston Children's Hospital reports that while cholesterol's "value to infants remains unclear . . . some experts have suggested it is necessary for the proper development of the nervous system." For that reason, and for others relating to overall health, the Hospital strongly recommends that *"cholesterol should not be restricted in the diet of infants, and only moderately restricted in young children's diets"* (emphasis theirs).

Lactose, the simple sugar in mother's milk, is readily converted in an infant's body to glucose, the brain's energy source. It has another quality that sets it apart from any sugar that's substituted for it in a formula. Absorbed slowly, it remains in the baby's intestine long enough to nurture those bacteria living there that benefit the infant in these ways: They fight off harmful bacteria; help in the absorption of minerals (including brain-vital calcium and magnesium); and manufacture B-complex vitamins, the group of vitamins most important in building the structures of the growing brain.

As they come to a child in mother's milk, the amino acids, the fats, cholesterol, and lactose, are packaged with substances (enzymes) for easy digestion. In a well-nourished mother, the milk is also vitamin/mineral–rich, enabling the digested food to follow perfect metabolic pathways to sites where it's needed in the growing body/brain. (Unfortunately, many American women are not well nourished, and babies fed on their milk, which is poor at least in vitamins C and folic acid and the mineral iron, must be supplemented.)

Your infant also gains from breastfeeding in three other extraordinary ways:

Immunoglobulins (IGs), proteins that form the first line of defense against many viruses and bacteria, are present in the "colostrum," the first fluid secreted by the breasts after birth. IGs protect the infant from a wide range of dangerous diseases including flu, pneumonia, whooping cough, diphtheria, "staph," polio, tetanus, salmonella, and gastroenteritis. In one study of 107 babies hospitalized for gastrointestinal disorders, 106 had not been breastfed.

Not only is mother's milk not allergenic, it contains a substance that blocks the action of allergens including brain allergens.

To blaze new pathways in the brain during the second birth of the baby's brain, stimulation is mandatory—and breastfeeding is the child's earliest stimulation, perhaps nature's way of starting and speeding the new brain growth. "Breast is best for a child's intellectual development," states Dr. Ralph Minear, "extremely important to the child's behavior and emotional development."

Dr. Miriam Stoppard, the renowned British expert on child care, adds experimental evidence. One group of laboratory monkeys, breastfed, grew up normally. The other group, bottle-fed, grew up "moody, aggressive, quarrelsome, pugnacious, and generally troublesome." Comments Dr. Stoppard: "Similar problems arise with human babies."

What should a woman eat during breastfeeding?

Your infant's nutritional demands are fundamentally the same as during pregnancy, and they are satisfied in the same way—with the high-fat/cholesterol diet recommended by Dr. Minear, fully ODA–vitamin/mineral supplemented. This is the basis for the breastfeeding program in our Eating Plan for Brighter Kids.

Can you benefit from breastfeeding?

In many ways.

It's great for your figure. Breastfeeding releases hormones that quickly dissipate pregnancy fat, and return to normal the size and contours of your uterus, pelvis, and waistline.

It could be a natural contraceptive. The hormone that produces breast milk, prolactin, also suppresses ovulation. (But your doctor is likely to tell you not to rely on this fact.)

Breastfeeding may act as a cancer-preventive. In many countries in which breastfeeding is the norm, there is less breast cancer than in the United States.

It can save you time and money. You don't have to prepare breast milk, buy equipment to make it, or make it.

It's dependable. "Infants are remarkably efficient at regulating their own diets," Boston Children's Hospital assures you. "When the baby is hungry, he or she makes this very clear." Wonderfully, *when* the baby makes this very clear, the breasts of a healthy mother naturally will have produced the right amount of milk to meet the demand. That's one reason many doctors recommend demand feeding to nursing mothers.

There is one benefit, though, that outshines all others. It's "bonding," a transcendent emotional experience that is uniquely a woman's. When an infant suckles, when it feels the nourishment—life, itself—flowing from you, and associates it with your closeness, your warmth, the perfume of your body, your touch, the light in your eyes, the embracing and the cuddling, a bond is forged that can enrich your life, and the life of your child, all your lives. It's the bond of love.

It's no wonder, then, that with all the natural benefits of breastfeeding, it has been the custom from time immemorial for mothers to keep their babies at their breasts until the babies, no longer needing mother's milk, reject it. That time, throughout history, has been about three years—a period corresponding to the major growth of the child's brain after its second birth.

But in this country today, a de facto deadline for terminating breastfeeding has been set at six months. Many women terminate even sooner. Of every 100 women who start breastfeeding in the hospital, only 75 continue to breastfeed after two months; and only 46 after five months. At six months, the number plummets to virtually zero. (And for every 100 mothers who breastfeed at all, there's another 100 who never do.)

But if mother's milk is the perfect food during the three years of the brain's second birth, how can kids be fed bright when they're deprived of it entirely or after six months at the most?

Feeding Your Kids to Brightness After Breastfeeding: The Mother's Milk Principle

The brilliantly simple solution came in 1983 from Dr. Ralph Minear of Harvard Medical School. He calls it the "Mother's Milk Principle," and in essence it's this: You can feed your kids bright without mother's milk when you replace it with a diet whose basic nutritional composition closely resembles mother's milk.

Rejecting baby formula as a mother's milk substitute—"No formula can compare with mother's milk, either for a baby's general dietary needs or for the specific requirements of a child's growing brain"—and recognizing the futility of attempting to replace mother's milk with any other food—"It's impossible to find any single sort of food that is the nutritional equivalent of breastfeeding for children up to 3 years of age'"—Dr. Minear advocates:

"For at least the first 3 years of life—and in modified form up to age 5—the proportions of carbohydrates, fats, and proteins in the diet of a young child should come as close as possible to those of breast milk. This means that fat in the child's daily calorie consumption should range up to 50 percent; complex carbohydrates should be 35 to 45 percent; and proteins . . . should be 8 to 15 percent." He observes, "In general, these values reflect what modern medical studies show to be the best brain food diet—and the best program for overall nutrition as well."

He defends the high-fat content of his diet—15 to 20 percent higher than in most doctor-recommended adult diets—saying, "Studies of the composition of human milk show it contains about 55 percent fats," and adding, "Now it's true that some physicians have expressed concern that atherosclerosis . . . from too high a fat content in the blood may begin at a . . . young age. But there have been no studies that show there is any danger of feeding very young children fats in accordance with the Mother's Milk Principle. The fact is, a child needs more fats . . . at least up to age 3 and probably up to age 5—largely because of the tremendous brain development that takes place during this time of life."

Whole milk, not skim milk, supplies these fats. For general health reasons, "young children need the fatty acids in whole milk," advises Boston Children's Hospital. "Skim milk is *not* better for children younger than two years old" (emphasis ours). At age 2, dendrites, essential to setting up connections between brain cells, reach their maximum number.

"Don't feed your preschooler an adult diet that is low in fats," Dr. Minear advises parents. "Rather, if you want to maximize your chances of increasing your child's brain power . . . *keep the distribution of fats up around 50 percent*" (emphasis his).

How do you feed your infant on the Mother's Milk Principle after *breast-feeding?*

This is how, based primarily on Dr. Minear's eating plan for infants, you can apply the Mother's Milk Principle to your baby's diet from 4 months to 1 year.

Months 4 and 5. During this time, you may introduce solid baby foods, although many doctors recommend 6 months as the starting date. But, cautions Boston Children's Hospital, do not begin before month 4. "Babies younger . . . are not developmentally ready for solid foods, and the agonies of such early feedings are wasted efforts because little food actually ends up in the baby."

Start with 1 to 2 teaspoons daily of an iron-fortified dry cereal mixed with breast milk (preferably) or formula. Increase the amount gradually to 2½ to 3 tablespoons twice a day. In addition, 6 breast-feedings are recommended in the fourth month, and 5 to 6 in the fifth. Your infant should suckle about 10 to 20 minutes at each breast. If your baby is on formula, five 5 to 8 ounce feedings daily is required in month 4, and five 6 to 8 ounce feedings in month 5.

You can begin with any cereal, but most pediatricians prefer iron-fortified rice cereal as baby's first solid, since it is the cereal most unlikely to cause an allergic reaction. After that, introduce barley, oatmeal, wheat, or high-protein cereal one at a time over five-day intervals so that an allergic reaction to a specific cereal can be spotted, and the offending food stricken from your baby's diet.

During month 4, the cereal mixes, which you prepared at first with a consistency only slightly less than that of breast milk or formula, is gradually thickened. By month 5, your baby is ready for the smooth, creamy texture of strained fruits and vegetables. You can use commercial baby foods, or you can prepare them yourself with a whir of the blender from some of the cooked fruits and vegetables on our Eating Plan for Brighter Kids. *"A baby's food should not be seasoned with salt or sugar,"* warns Boston Children's Hospital (emphasis theirs); and on our basic eating Plan, there's not a grain of sugar, and no salt or extremely small amounts that can be eliminated. (In the "goiter belt," though, some iodized salt may be advisable. Consult your pediatrician.) Actually, most of the solid food for your baby from months 4 to 12 can be derived from that Plan.

Months 6 to 8. In the sixth month, for most breast-fed babies, bottle-fed formula is introduced and, for most babies, strained foods give way gradually to finely mashed ("junior-texture") foods.

Should you delay this textural upgrading by a month or two, your baby may attempt to stay at the strained-food level even longer, lengthening the time a baby normally takes to eat regular family-textured foods (about 10 months to one year). A baby that has become accustomed to finely mashed foods in the sixth month, happily begins the transition to minced foods in the seventh.

During months 6 to 8, Dr. Minear recommends each day iron-enriched formula, cereal, vegetables, and fruit. He prefers that you serve your baby *"five meals a day and limit each serving of a solid to four tablespoons"* (emphasis his). Dr. Minear bases his five-meal preference essentially on "studies [that] have demonstrated . . . nutrients are best utilized . . . in the body in small amounts, rather than in large, infrequent servings." (Some pediatricians favor demand feedings up to seven months; others approve of starting infants on three meals a day in the sixth month. Your pediatrician should be your guide.)

In the sixth month, your baby's gustatory horizon is broadening. Now the menu of finely mashed fruits and vegetables, according to Dr. Spock, can include pineapples, string beans, squash, onions, asparagus, chard, and tomatoes. Many pediatricians add finely mashed macaroni, spaghetti, and noodles to that list. Soft ripe bananas, fork-mashed, get a nod of approval from Boston Children's Hospital.

But warning signs are up: Avoid broccoli, cauliflower, cabbage, and sweet potatoes, warns Dr. Spock. Dr. Minear tells you to eliminate onions and cucumbers. Nutritionist Miriam Erick, who specializes in developing intelligent eating techniques for mother and child, forbids corn, lima beans, and plain yogurt. All nutrition scientists agree that infants' intestines, unlike older kids', are vulnerable to toxic botulism spores that may appear in some honeys; so honey and foods containing it are outlawed for children under age 1.

Around the seventh month, your baby enjoys the first tastes of finely minced food, as chicken, lamb, liver, veal, and pork replace some of the cereal. Potatoes and pasta, finely minced, are also a delightful new experience. This is teething time, and hard toast and crackers help soothe the discomfort.

Perhaps the greatest joy of your infant's adventures in eating comes between the seventh and tenth months when finger foods are encountered. These are small pieces of food that challenge the baby's growing ability to pick up things with thumb and forefinger. Gastronomically, they range from soft baby-sized bits of cheese, ripe fresh fruit (peeled and seed-free), and steamed vegetables (no ends, strings and peels) to tofu cubes, mini-meatballs, and tiny slices of boneless and skinless tenderly cooked chicken and fish. Fun for infants, who treat these bright-hued morsels as toys—edible toys—they stir your child's brain, and are part of the food-stimulation mechanism of brain growth that began when you first took your baby to your breast.

Months 8 to 10. Dr. Minear's daily eating plan for this period calls for iron-fortified formula, juice, vegetables, fruits, meats, fish, yogurt, cheese, cooked dried beans, peanut butter, and egg yolk. Egg yolk is an excellent source of brain-needed cholesterol. But egg whites, which may be allergens to some infants up to 10 months, are banned; as are egg-white-containing foods such as ice cream.

In the eighth month, your child is learning how to drink from a cup. Whole milk, not skim, replaces some of the formula. Mild spices delight the palate; and by the ninth month, the texture of chopped foods adds a new joy. If your child had been demand-fed up to the seventh month, the regime of three meals a day and snacks, begun then, has become fairly routine. You're delighted with the progress your baby is making toward eating family foods with the whole family.

Months 10 to 12. On Dr. Minear's eating plan, your baby is still on iron-fortified formula; but there's less of it. To that is added each day cereal, bread, fruit, vegetables, plain yogurt, 1 whole egg; peanut butter, cooked dried beans, meat, fish, chicken, and fruit juice.

By the end of the twelfth month, your baby has been fed, Dr. Minear says, "the sort of food a baby needs to enhance . . . maximum brain growth in the first year of life." And for the years to come? At age 1, your baby has been weaned, and has taken a place at the family table, sharing the family's food. But how can you meet adults' needs and children's needs with the same menu plan? How can you feed the grown-ups right and your kids' bright with the same meals?

The answer, which follows, comes from the food/brightness revolution in the kitchen.

The Nutrition/
Brightness Revolution
in the Kitchen:
The Eating Plan for
Brighter Kids

11

SELECTING YOUR KIDS' FOODS

The 181 Worst Foods for Your Kids' Brains; The 265 Best Foods for Your Kids' Brains

This part of the book is your operating manual for our Eating Plan for Brighter Kids. It tells you precisely what to do to feed your kids to brightness.

It starts, in this chapter, with a group of foods to eliminate from your kitchen, and a group of foods to put on your "must" list.

Then, in subsequent chapters, it provides you with instructions for:

- setting up an easily do-able menu plan for brightness

- getting rid of the junk-food habit in an utterly different and delicious way

- learning how to create a four-star menu with our new "bright cuisine"

- eating right to feed your kids bright during pregnancy and breastfeeding

- serving your kids the brightest foods from age 1 to adolescence

- selecting the right vitamin/mineral supplements for yourself during preconception, pregnancy, and breastfeeding; and for your kids, starting at age 2

The remarkable thing about this Eating Plan for Brighter Kids is that it's a single healthful program for the whole family, simply modified for your special needs and your kids'.

What the "Worst" and "Best" Food Lists Are All About

A junk food is vitamin/mineral–impoverished, providing little support for kids' (and adults') bodies and brains. It's also rife with harmful ingredients that attack the body/brain and to which kids are especially vulnerable. These are sugar, salt and other sodium compounds, saturated fats, chemical colorings, flavorings, preservatives, stimulants, processing ingredients, and other additives.

A junk food is, for example, this mix: sugar (sucrose), nonfat milk solids, corn syrup solids, cream, whole milk, guar gum, sodium hexametaphosphate, carrageenan, salt, imitation vanilla powder, sodium alginate, cellulose gum, dextrose, and F.D.& C. yellow dyes Nos. 5 and 6. Recognize it? It's a "milk shake" served in fast-food shops, and, unfortunately, still in many school lunchrooms.

But some natural foods are as bad as junk foods—robbing children's brains of nutrients, impeding the brain's functions, and sometimes actually destroying the brain's tissues. They could make your kids hyperactive or slow learners; turn them into Jekyll-and-Hydes; slash their I.Q.'s; brown out their brains; and produce a startling catalog of mental, emotional, behavioral, and learning problems.

The most harmful of natural foods, and the most harmful of junk foods, have here been assembled for the first time in the 181 Worst Foods for Your Kids' Brains. Take the list into your kitchen, and if any of the items are on your shelves or in your fridge (they are), get rid of them today and never trundle them to the check-out counter again.

Instead, from now on make your food selections mainly from the 265 Best Foods for Your Kids' Brains. Fresh foods with the highest of nutrient contents, and a sprinkling of processed foods of exceptional value, they provide the soundest foundation for the health of your kids' brains and for the general health of the whole family.

They're familiar foods, many are among America's longtime favorites—*and* there's no need to go out of your way to get them. It seems unbelievable, but it's true: The road to your children's brightness begins in the supermarket.

One final incentive for making the switch from the worst foods to the best foods for your kids' brains: Foods work on kids' brains fast. You could see results in just a few weeks. Or sooner.

The 181 Worst Foods for Your Kids' Brains

• ———————————— •

This is your guide to what foods to pass by as you wheel your cart from department to department in your supermarket. These foods should be eliminated on adults' as well as children's diets because, as a group, they are high in sugar and salt, contain excessive amounts of cholesterol and fats—all associated by nutrition scientists with adult degenerative diseases such as heart attack, diabetes, and cancer. All the products listed here are "commercial." **Asterisked (*) items** are foods that inhibit the action of some vitamins and minerals in the body/brain; but they can be used on a fully supplemented diet. For specific lists of foods that may trigger hyperactivity, brain allergies, goiter, and brain brown-outs in some children, see Chapters 2, 3, 5, and 6/8 respectively. A list of high-fiber foods, which when consumed in excess may harm some children's brains, is found in Chapter 8.

Baked Goods

Bagels
Baking powder*
Baking soda*
Brioches
Brownies
Cakes and crackers
Cookies
Corn bread
Croissants
Dietetic bread
Doughnuts
Gluten bread
Pastries
Pies
Pumpernickel
Rolls
Rye bread
Salt sticks
Swedish flat breads
Sweet rolls
White bread
Zwiebach

Beverages

Alcoholic beverages
Chocolate milk
Cocoa
Coffee
Diet drinks
Fruit-type drinks
Instant drinks
Soft drinks,
    including cola drinks
Tea (including most herb
    teas)

The 181 Worst Foods for Your Kids' Brains (cont.)

•————————•

Breakfast Foods

Bacon
Granola
Ham

High-sugar breakfast cereals
Sausages

Canned, Frozen, and Instant Foods

Baking mixes
Bouillon-type cubes
Canned entrées
Canned fruits
Canned juices
Canned soups
Canned vegetables
Dessert mixes
Frozen baked foods

Frozen prepared
  foods and meals
Frozen uncooked foods
Instant breakfast mixes
Powdered drink mixes
Prepared stuffings
Sauce mixes
Seasoning mixes
Soup mixes

(Exceptions in this category are canned salt-, sugar- and additives-free products when used on a fully supplemented diet.)

Condiments, Sauces, Salad Dressings

Chili sauce
Chutney
Horseradish
Ketchup
Mayonnaise
Prepared mustards

Salad dressings, packaged
  and bottled
Soy and other Oriental
  sauces
Steak sauces
Tabasco

Cooked Take-outs

Barbecued poultry
French fries
Fried chicken

Fried fish
Hamburgers
Rotisseried chicken

Dairy Products

Coffee whiteners
Dessert whips, synthetic
Egg whites*
Flavored yogurts

High-fat cheeses (such as
  Brie, Gruyère, Muenster,
  and Gorgonzola)
Processed cheeses

Delicatessen

Bologna
Coleslaw
Fish salads
Frankfurters
German-type wursts
  (including liverwurst)
Italian-type cold cuts
  (including prosciutto)
Luncheon meats

Meat salads
Olives
Pastrami
Pickled vegetables
  (including "pickles")
Pickles
Salami
Sauerkraut
Vegetable salads

Desserts

Candy
Chocolate
Custards
Flavored gelatin
Fruit toppings
Ice cream
Ice milk
Ices

Jams
Jellies
Junket desserts
Mousses
Puddings
Sherbets
Syrups

Fats and Oils

Artificially colored butter
  (except if colored with
  beta-carotene, which is
  beneficial)
Coconut oil

Hardened white vegetable
  shortenings (hydrogenated
  vegetable fats)
Margarine (with additives)
Lard and other animal fats
Palm oil

The 181 Worst Foods for Your Kids' Brains (cont.)

•────────────•

Fish

Caviar and other roes
Fillets, preserved in brine
  and/or artificially colored
Fish, raw*
Fish sticks
Red snapper (may be high in
  toxic mercury)

Smoked fish (including
  Scotch salmon, Nova
  Scotia salmon, Norwegian
  salmon, finnan haddie)

Meats and Poultry

Capon
Duck
Fatty cuts of meat
Goose
Kidneys

Lungs
Roaster chicken
Self-basting poultry
Sweetbreads

Produce

Almonds*
Avocados
Beets, raw*
Cabbage, raw
Cassava*
Cauliflower*
Coconut
Corn and corn products*
  (except corn oil)
Horseradish*
Kale*

Mustard greens
Piñon (female pine-seed)
  nuts
Rape
Rutabaga*
Soy beans and soy bean
  products*
Spinach, raw*
Turnips, raw*
Vegetable greens, raw*
Watercress*

Snacks

Cheese puffs
  and similar snack items
Creme-filled baked goods
Dips
Granola bars
Peanuts
Popcorn

Potato chips
Pretzels
Salted nuts
Seeds*
Snack-type fruit pies
Walnuts, Persian*

Sugars and Sugar Substitutes

Aspartame
Beet sugar
Blackstrap molasses
Brown sugar
Cane sugar
Corn syrup
Dextrins
Dextrose
Equal
Fructose
Glucose
HFCS (high fructose corn
  syrup)
Honey, processed; or any
  for kids under age 1

Inert sugar
Mannitol
Maple syrup
NutraSweet
Pancake syrups
Raw sugar
Saccharin
Sorbitol
Sucrose (table sugar)
Turbinado sugar
Yellow-D
Xylitol

The 265 Best Foods for Your Kids' Brains

• ——————————————— •

These are the foods with the highest obtainable nutrient content. The best possible foods for meeting the needs of your kids' bodies and brains, they're also the best possible foods for adult health needs. As a group, they're low in saturated fats and cholesterol, contain no added sugar and salt, and supply the right amount of fiber—all factors in warding off nutrition-related diseases. (The higher optimal amounts of fats and cholesterol needed by children from conception to at least ages 3 to 5 are provided for in our Eating Plan for Brighter Kids by menu planning.)

The foods are arranged here in Food Groups, not the traditional four or five, but an easier-to-use eleven—one major result of the nutrition revolution in the kitchen. By selecting servings from each food group according to a simple formula (Chapter 15), you can obtain the best possible nutritional mix for your children and the adults in your family. All foods are natural and fresh by modern standards, with the exceptions of a few acceptable processed foods. **Asterisked (*) items** are permitted only on a fully supplemented diet.

Food Group 1
ANIMAL FOODS/EGGS

Eggs

Fish (Fish oils—an oil is a liquid fat—are polyunsaturated, the type of oil that fights nutrition-related diseases such as heart attack, diabetes, and cancer.)

Low Fat

Abalone	Pike
Cod	Pollock
Flounder	Sea bass (white)
Gray snapper	Scrod
Haddock	Skate
Hake	Sole
Perch (yellow)	Tilefish

Moderate Fat

Albacore	Porgy
Barracuda (Pacific)	Redfish (ocean perch)
Bass (all varieties except sea	Salmon, pink
bass)	Smelt
Bluefish	Sturgeon
Carp	Swordfish
Catfish	Trout, brook
Halibut	Tuna
Herring	Whiting
Monkfish	

Meat*

(These are lean cuts when purchased as "choice" rather than "prime." The fats are saturated, the type associated with nutrient-related diseases. Excess should be avoided. Even in small quantities saturated fats may not be metabolized properly without full vitamin/mineral supplementation. Chemical-free meat is recommended.)

Beef

Chuck steak	Roast beef (round)
Double-bone sirloin	Rump
Filet mignon	Shell steak
Flank steak	Short plate
London broil	Sirloin steak
Porterhouse	T-bone steak

Lamb (leanest cuts in choice)

Leg	Shoulder chops
Loin chops and other loin	Rib chops
cuts	

Pork (leanest cuts in choice)
Fresh ham
Picnic pork

Rabbit

The 265 Best Foods for Your Kids' Brains (cont.)

• ──────────────── •

Veal (leanest cuts in choice)
Leg   Round
Loin chops and other loin   Rump
   cuts   Shoulder chops

Venison

Poultry

Chicken   Squab
   Fryer, light or dark meat   Turkey
Cornish hen   (young, light or dark
Pheasant   meat)
Quail

Seafood

Crab   Mussels
Clams   Oyster
Crayfish   Scallops
Lobster   Shrimp

Food Group 2
MILK/YOGURT/CHEESE

Milk (Buttermilk, nonfat, and skim for adults and adolescents; whole milk for pregnant and nursing mothers, and children up to age 5, at least)

Buttermilk   Skim milk
Dry milk   Whole milk
   Nonfat dry milk
   Whole dry milk

Yogurt (see Milk)

Plain low-fat yogurt
Plain whole-milk yogurt

Cheese (nonprocessed)

Cottage cheese

Farmer cheese

Mozzarella

Parmesan

Pot cheese

Ricotta

Food Group 3
GRAINS

Barley

Millet

Old-fashioned rolled oats

Regular Cream of Wheat

Regular wheat germ

Rice

Wheat flakes

Whole kasha (buckwheat
   groats)

Wild rice

Food Group 4
BREAD/CRACKERS/INGREDIENTS

Arrowroot flour

Baking soda*

Buckwheat flour

Cornstarch

Double-acting baking
   powder, without
   aluminum*

Dry yeast

Pasta (preferably made from
   flour and water, no salt or
   other additives,
   Neapolitan style, like
   spaghetti, macaroni, and
   linguine)

Rye flour

Stone-ground whole-wheat
   flour

Unbleached flour

Whole-wheat pastry flour

Food Group 5
LEGUMES/NUTS/SEEDS

All nuts (especially walnuts,
   but almonds,* peanuts*
   and Persian walnuts* only
   on a fully supplemented
   diet)

All nut butters, see previous
   listing

Dried beans

Dried peas (including split
   peas and chick-peas)

Lentils

Sesame seeds

Sunflower seeds

Tofu (bean curd)*

The 265 Best Foods for Your Kids' Brains (cont.)

• ────────────── •

Food Group 6
VITAMIN-C FRUITS/VEGETABLES

Fruits

Black cherry concentrate
Cantaloupe
Grapefruit
Guava
Honeydew melon
Juices (fresh; frozen only on
    a fully supplemented diet)
Limes
Mango
Orange
Papaya
Lemons
Pineapple
Strawberries
Tangerine

Vegetables

Broccoli
Cauliflower*
Green pepper
Parsnips
Peas
Pea pods
Potatoes
Rhubarb
Sprouts
Squash (summer/winter)
Sweet potatoes
Sweet red pepper
Tomatoes †
Tomato juice †
Tomato paste †
Tomato puree †
Vegetable juices †
Zucchini

† Canned, only with no salt added, on a fully supplemented diet

Food Group 7
DARK GREEN VEGETABLES

Asparagus
Broccoli
Brussels sprouts*
Cabbage (cooked)
Chard
Dark leafy lettuce
Escarole
Red leaf lettuce
Romaine lettuce
Scallions

Chicory

Chinese cabbage (bok choy)

Endive

Spinach (cooked)

Turnip (cooked)

Watercress*

Food Group 8

OTHER FRUITS/VEGETABLES

Fruits

Apples

Apricots

Bananas

Blueberries

Cherries

Cranberries

Dates

Figs

Grapes

Juices (fresh; frozen only on
a fully supplemented diet)

Nectarines

Peaches

Pears

Plums

Prunes

Raisins

Raspberries

Vegetables

Artichoke

Bamboo shoots

Beets (cooked)

Carrots

Celery

Corn*

Corn for popping*

Cucumber

Eggplant

Green beans

Mushrooms

Okra

Onions

Pumpkin

Radishes

Yams

Food Group 9

FATS

Cold-pressed vegetable oils

Corn oil

Cottonseed oil

Peanut oil

Safflower oil

Sesame oil (not Oriental
variety)

Soybean oil

Sunflower oil

Virgin olive oil

Walnut oil

The 265 Best Foods for Your Kids' Brains (cont.)

•———————————•

Butter, sweet (no salt)

(natural, or colored only
  with beta-carotene, which
  is beneficial)

Food Group 10
SWEETS

Carob powder and chips
  (unsweetened)
Date powder
Dried fruits (unprocessed)
Fruit juices (fresh; frozen
  only on a fully
  supplemented diet)
Honey (uncooked,
  unfiltered; not for
  children under
  age 1)
Nuts (raw), see under "All
  nuts" in *Food Group 5*

Nut pastes (no sugar or salt
  added), see previous
  listing
Sugar cane
Sweet herbs (aniseed,
  marjoram, oregano,
  rosemary, sweet basil,
  tarragon)
Sweet spices (allspice,
  cinnamon, coriander,
  ginger, mace, sweet
  paprika)

Food Group 11
HERBS/SPICES/CONDIMENTS/FLAVORINGS

Regarded until recently by conventional medical sciences as
nonnutritive, herbs and spices are now known, thanks mainly
to comprehensive chemical analyses conducted by the U.S. Department of Agriculture (USDA), to be replete with essential
vitamins and minerals. They may also contribute substances
that fight destructive biochemicals (oxidants and their deriva-
tives) that attack all cells in the body, including the brain's. We
use both fresh and dried herbs.

Garlic is not only the most nutritionally potent food in this
group (it *is* an herb), but, used judiciously, it can also be a

culinary delight. There's widening acceptance by conventional doctors of this popular herb's preventive medical properties.

Herbs/Spices

Allspice
Aniseed
Basil or sweet basil
Bay leaves
Caraway seeds
Cardamom seeds
Cayenne (red pepper)
Chervil
Chili con carne seasoning (no salt added)
Chives
Cinnamon
Cloves
Coriander seeds
Cumin
Curry powder (no salt added)
Dill
Fennel seeds
Garlic
Ginger
Juniper berries
Mace
Marjoram
Mustard seeds
Nutmeg
Onion powder (not onion salt)
Oregano
Parsley
Pickling spices (no salt added)
Poppy seeds
Rosemary
Sage
Savory
Shallots
Tarragon
Thyme
Watercress

Condiments/Flavorings

Apple cider vinegar
Balsamic vinegar
Grain coffee (also called cereal beverage; not a coffee, but has a coffeelike flavor as an adult drink; as used as a flavoring in my recipes, it does not taste like coffee)
Low-sodium vegetable seasoning
Pure vanilla extract
Reduced-sodium soy sauce
Smoked yeast
Vanilla bean
Wine vinegar

12

HASSLE-FREE MEALS FOR BRIGHTER KIDS

The Basic All-Family Menu Plan

This is as healthful a basic family eating plan as can be created based on the most up-to-date medical information on the total health needs of adults and children. The plan follows the basic dietary principles of the American Medical Association, the Federal Dietary Guidelines for Americans, the American Dietetic Association, and the American Academy of Pediatrics, and incorporates the discoveries of the nutrition/brightness revolutions.

It's a menu plan designed for health-conscious cooks in a hurry. Kitchen time has been shrunk to a minimum; it's cooking-simple; and shopping is supermarket-easy.

Yet there's been no loss in taste appeal. Swift, transforming touches do wonders with the simplest of dishes—sandwiches, salads, omelettes, chicken, hot cereals, spreads, tuna—even fruits and vegetables. Your kids won't be able to wait for the next servings of Sautéed Bananas or Sautéed Oriental Mix of vegetables, and neither will you or your husband. There's even a new exciting snack treat for the whole family, a Peanut Butter Milk Shake, that takes almost no time to make.

The Basic All-Family Menu Plan uses mainly those foods listed on the 265 Best Foods for Your Kids' Brains. They've been combined to supply the best possible quantities of nutrients in the most beneficial proportions by making selections from the eleven Food Groups, according to our adaptation of a formula developed by Alice White. A brilliant innovator who helped create the nutritional revolution in the kitchen, Alice White has been a nutritionist for the Federal Maternal Infants and Children's Care Program and a nutrition consultant to the Harvard School of Public Health.

Low in saturated fats and cholesterol, stingy with salt, containing virtually no sugar, moderate in fiber, with all the essential amino acids and just the right amount of calories, and without a trace of "worst foods," this is the ideal menu plan for men and nonpregnant women. It can be easily adapted with just minor modifications for you during pregnancy and breastfeeding, and for your kids up to age 5 (that's in Chapter 15).

But at no time will you be making meals for yourself, meals for your husband, and meals for your kids. You'll be making a single meal for all, and just altering portion sizes and adding or subtracting a few ingredients to meet the special needs of your kids and yourself.

The Basic All-Family Menu Plan is a model. Use it as-is, or spin off on your own variations by replacing any food with a similar Best-265 Food from the same Food Group. You can, for example, replace "orange sections," a member of Food Group 6, Vitamin-C Fruits/Vegetables, with any of thirteen different fruits. This simple replacement technique helps you create an almost endless variety of menus. The Basic All-Family Menu Plan is an exciting, never boring, healthful eating program.

But if you meet wistful resistance from the junk-food lovers among you—including yourself—go to the next chapter and learn how to break the junk-food habit by including any of more than sixty "junk foods" in the Basic All-Family Menu Plan. But the wonderful thing about these junk foods is that they taste like junk foods, they look like junk foods, they're named like junk foods, but they're not junk foods at all. They're healthful "junk-food" clones.

And if you long for that four-star gourmet touch—and we think it's wonderful if you do, because what a gift you'll be giving your kids by introducing them to the joys of the great tastes of food, healthful food—go to Chapter 14 and learn how you can make our new "Bright Cuisine" replacements on the Basic Menus.

The Basic All-Family Menu Plan, and its healthful "junk-food" and Bright Cuisine variants, are easily adapted to your special needs during pregnancy and breastfeeding, and the needs of your kids from infancy to adolescence. Find out how to do it in Chapter 15. (For example, skim milk in the menus that follow is replaced with whole milk for young kids.)

When should you start your family on the Basic All-Family Menu Plan?

Tomorrow.

At breakfast.

The Basic All-Family Menu Plan
• ——————————————— •

Before you begin, keep these notes in mind:

- The term *homemade* in the following menus means your own recipe prepared with minimum salt and with no sugar.
- For an after-meal drink, for adults only, grain coffee (also called cereal beverage) is a caffeine-free coffee taste-alike. But it's not for kids; you don't want them to get used to the taste of coffee. Water is a great drink; many of us have forgotten how good it is.
- Oil and vinegar dressing is made with one part any vinegar and two parts vegetable oil.
- Butter or margarine for kids? Margarine is lower in saturated fats, higher in polyunsaturated fats, and contains no cholesterol—all of which contributes to preventing cardiovascular problems and heart attack. This is fine for adults and children over age 5. But children under that age need cholesterol for the growth and functioning of the nervous system and the I.Q.-related glial-cell complex in the brain; and butter is an excellent source of cholesterol. We compromise by using a butter-margarine blend. Boston Children's Hospital advises that instead of purchasing a commercial combination, it's "easy and more economical to soften a stick of each and blend them together at home." Sweet butter (unsalted) without artificial coloring (except beta-carotene, which is beneficial) is the best of the butters; and margarine should be free of additives (except beta-carotene). Switching your over-age-5 children to margarine may be beneficial. There is no difference in calories between butter and regular margarine; but "diet margarine," which contains more water, is less caloric.
- In addition to selections from The 265 Best Foods, we also include some variants (like evaporated skim milk) and some of the rehabilitated junk foods (page 75).
- Do remember that this Basic All-Family Menu Plan is just that —the *base* for getting started—on which you can build your own exciting menus which include "junk food" clones and gourmet Bright Cuisine dishes.

• ———————— DAY 1 ———————— •

BREAKFAST

¾ cup low-fat plain yogurt, mixed with fresh orange sections *or* ½ cup berries in season
1 scrambled egg, prepared with:
  • 1 teaspoon sweet butter/margarine blend
  • dash each curry powder and dried tarragon leaves, crushed
2 slices whole-wheat bread
1 tablespoon unsweetened jelly
1 cup skim milk

LUNCH

1 cup homemade tomato soup *or* low-sodium tomato juice served with homemade unsalted popcorn
1 tuna salad sandwich, prepared with:
  • 3 ounces canned tuna packed in water
  • 1 tablespoon each chopped onion and celery
  • 2 teaspoons fresh lemon juice
  • 1 teaspoon Italian olive oil
  • 2 slices whole-wheat bread
1 fresh pear *or* apple

DINNER

¼ small chicken, skinned, broiled or roasted, rubbed all over with 1 teaspoon oil, and sprinkled with:
  • ⅛ teaspoon each mild paprika and onion powder
  • ¼ teaspoon dried sage leaves
  • pinch salt (optional)
1 medium baked yam or sweet potato
½ cup steamed broccoli, sprinkled with fresh lemon juice
1 small sliced tomato, surrounded with:
  • julienned sweet green pepper
  • shredded carrot
  • radish roses
  • 1 tablespoon oil and vinegar dressing
½ cup fresh pineapple cubes, or canned crushed pineapple packed in unsweetened pineapple juice
1 cup skim milk

• ——————————— DAY 2 ——————————— •

BREAKFAST

1 cup grapefruit and orange sections, sweetened with:
  • 1 teaspoon honey, dissolved in
  • 2 tablespoons unsweetened apple juice
½ cup hot oatmeal *or* Cream of Wheat seasoned with:
  • dash salt
  • ⅛ teaspoon ground cinnamon
  • 1 teaspoon honey
2 slices whole-wheat bread
1 teaspoon sweet butter/margarine blend
1 tablespoon unsweetened jelly *or* unsweetened fruit butter
1 cup skim milk

LUNCH

1 cup homemade mushroom and barley soup
1 sliced chicken or turkey sandwich, prepared with:
  • 2 slices whole-wheat bread
  • spread composed of ½ teaspoon each tomato paste, olive oil,
    and prepared Dijon mustard
  • 2 ounces sliced chicken or turkey (do not use chicken or turkey
    roll)
1 medium tomato, sliced, topped with crisp alfalfa sprouts
½ cup homemade applesauce sweetened with honey
1 cup skim milk

DINNER

3 ounces grilled veal patty, *or* sliced London broil, seasoned with
  herbs and spices
1 cup spaghetti or macaroni with homemade tomato sauce *or* salt/
  sugar-free commercial sauce, sprinkled with:
  • minced fresh herbs
  • ½ teaspoon freshly grated Parmesan cheese
½ cup steamed green beans, sprinkled with:
  • freshly grated nutmeg
  • lemon juice
¼ small cantaloupe, ½ cup fresh berries in season, *or* ¼ cup raisin-
  nut mix
1 cup skim milk

——————— DAY 3 ———————

BREAKFAST

½ cup stewed fruit compote, topped with:
- • 1 tablespoon low-fat cottage cheese, and
- • 2 tablespoons undiluted evaporated skim milk (it's sweet tasting and good)

1 shredded wheat biscuit, sprinkled with 1 tablespoon date powder or regular wheat germ

1 cup skim milk

1 slice whole-wheat bread

½ teaspoon sweet butter/margarine blend

1 to 2 teaspoons unsweetened jelly

LUNCH

1 cup low-sodium V-8 *or* tomato juice

1 serving *Oriental Sauté*, prepared in wok or nonstick skillet with:
- • 2 teaspoons hot peanut oil
- • 1½ cups combined thinly sliced scallion, sweet red or green pepper, snow peas, and broccoli florets
- • 3 ounces cubed tofu (bean curd), dried on paper toweling
- • 1 teaspoon reduced-sodium soy sauce
- • 2 to 3 tablespoons homemade chicken broth, or broth made with low-sodium vegetable seasoning

½ cup cooked brown rice

¾ cup cubed fresh pineapple, *or* unsweetened pineapple chunks topped with 1 tablespoon unsalted peanut butter

1 cup skim milk

DINNER

3 ounces baked fresh fillet of scrod *or* flounder, prepared with:
- • 1½ teaspoons sweet butter/margarine blend
- • 1 teaspoon minced fresh dill or parsley
- • dash salt

½ cup steamed fresh peas

1 medium baked Idaho potato, split and topped with:
- • 1 tablespoon low-fat plain yogurt
- • 1 tablespoon minced chives

1 slice whole-wheat bread

½ teaspoon sweet butter/margarine blend

DAY 3 (*continued*)

¾ cup mixed salad, prepared with:
- ¼ cup each thinly sliced cucumber or zucchini, carrot, and mushrooms
- 1 tablespoon minced onion, *or* 1 scallion, coarsely chopped
- 1 tablespoon oil and vinegar dressing

1 medium banana, sliced and quickly sautéed in nonstick skillet with:
- 1 teaspoon sweet butter/margarine blend
- ¼ teaspoon each ground ginger and cinnamon
- 1 teaspoon fresh lemon juice (squeezed over cooked banana)

— DAY 4 —

BREAKFAST

1 whole orange, *or* ½ cup berries in season
½ cup Cream of Wheat prepared with:
  • 2 teaspoons unprocessed bran
  • dash each ground cinnamon and cardamom
  • 2 teaspoons honey
2 slices whole-wheat bread
1 teaspoon sweet butter/margarine blend
1 tablespoon unsweetened jelly
1 cup skim milk

LUNCH

1 cup homemade lentil soup
1 roast beef sandwich, prepared with:
  • 3 ounces lean roast beef
  • 2 slices whole-wheat bread
  • spread composed of ½ teaspoon each tomato paste, olive oil,
    and prepared Dijon mustard
  • freshly ground pepper (optional)
½ cup homemade applesauce sweetened with honey, *or* ¼ cup
  dried fruit, without preservatives
1 cup skim milk

DINNER

2 small chicken legs (skinned), *or* 4 ounces boned and skinned
  chicken breasts, first lightly browned in 1½ teaspoons corn oil,
  then sautéed with:
  • ½ teaspoon minced garlic
  • 1 tablespoon minced shallot
  • 2 tablespoons coarsely chopped sweet green or red pepper
  • 1 coarsely chopped egg tomato
  • 2 dashes salt
  then cooked, covered, over low heat until tender
½ cup steamed sliced carrots, sprinkled with pinch freshly grated
  nutmeg
½ cup cooked brown rice, sprinkled with minced fresh rosemary,
  dill, or parsley

DAY 4 (*continued*)

1 cup cut-up fresh fruit, *or* ¼ cup dried fruit, without preservatives
1 cup skim milk

DAY 5

BREAKFAST

½ broiled grapefruit, spooned before broiling with:
  - 1 teaspoon honey
  - 2 tablespoons unsweetened apple juice
3 whole wheat pancakes, prepared from scratch in nonstick skillet lightly coated with oil, batter mixed with skim milk (or a mixture of half skim and half whole milk)
1 tablespoon unsweetened jelly
1 cup skim milk

LUNCH

1 cup homemade chicken soup with noodles or rice
1 heated pita bread pocket, filled with layers of:
  - ¼ cup each cooked warm pinto beans and warm brown rice
  - 1 coarsely chopped egg tomato
  - 1 coarsely chopped hard-cooked egg, and sprinkled with
  - 1 tablespoon minced fresh parsley, dill, or rosemary
  - dash salt
1 cup skim milk

DINNER

1 cup low-sodium V-8 *or* tomato juice
1 3-ounce serving homemade beef or veal stew
½ cup cooked bulgur, sprinkled with:
  - ½ teaspoon minced shallot
  - 1 teaspoon minced fresh parsley, dill, or rosemary
½ cup steamed baby onions, seasoned with:
  - ½ teaspoon sweet butter/margarine blend
  - dash each salt and freshly grated nutmeg
1 serving zucchini salad, consisting of:
  - ¼ cup each alfalfa sprouts, grated carrot, and zucchini
  - julienne strips sweet red pepper
  - 1 tablespoon oil and vinegar dressing
¼ small cantaloupe, *or* ¼ cup raisin-nut mix
1 cup skim milk

DAY 6

BREAKFAST

1 medium baked apple, prepared with:
  • 2 tablespoons unsweetened pineapple or apple juice
  • 1 teaspoon honey (optional)
  • ¼ teaspoon ground cinnamon
  • dash ground ginger
1 open-faced cottage cheese sandwich, made with:
  • 2 slices whole-wheat bread
  • ½ cup low-fat cottage cheese, sprinkled with
  • 1 tablespoon regular wheat germ
1 cup skim milk

LUNCH

1 3-ounce hamburger, prepared with:
  • 2 slices whole-wheat bread
  • spread composed of ½ teaspoon each tomato paste, olive oil, and prepared Dijon mustard
  • thinly sliced onion
1 serving mixed vegetable salad, consisting of:
  • 1 coarsely chopped egg tomato
  • 1 small sliced Kirby cucumber
  • 4 sliced radishes
  • 1 tablespoon oil and vinegar dressing
  • ½ teaspoon freshly grated Parmesan cheese
½ cup fresh pineapple cubes, *or* canned crushed pineapple packed in unsweetened pineapple juice
1 cup skim milk

DINNER

1 cup homemade split pea soup, *or* low-sodium tomato juice
3 ounces broiled fresh salmon, *or* 5 fresh shrimp, prepared with:
  • 1 teaspoon sweet butter/margarine blend
  • ¼ teaspoon dried crushed tarragon leaves
  • dash each salt and pepper
  • fresh lemon juice

½ cup mashed potatoes, prepared with:
- 2 teaspoons low-fat plain yogurt
- 1 tablespoon chopped chives
- ⅛ teaspoon curry powder
- dash each salt and pepper

½ cup steamed fresh snow peas, seasoned with:
- ½ teaspoon sweet butter/margarine blend
- ⅛ teaspoon freshly grated nutmeg
- ¼ teaspoon apple cider vinegar
- dash each salt and pepper

1 fresh pear, *or* medium slice of watermelon
1 cup skim milk

• ───────────── **DAY 7** ───────────── •

BREAKFAST

½ cup stewed dried fruit compote (see Breakfast, DAY 3), *or* whole
   orange
 1 Western omelette, prepared in nonstick skillet with:
   • ½ teaspoon sweet butter/margarine blend
   • 1 beaten egg
   make filling in skillet with:
   • 1 teaspoon Italian olive oil
   • ¼ cup each chopped sweet green pepper, onion, and tomato
   • ¼ teaspoon crushed dried oregano leaves
   • ½ teaspoon smoked yeast
 2 slices whole-wheat bread
 1 cup skim milk

LUNCH

 1 cup homemade gazpacho *or* tomato soup
 1 sardine sandwich, prepared with:
   • 3 ounces Norwegian sardines packed in water
   • 1 tablespoon chopped scallion or onion
   • 1 teaspoon fresh lemon juice
   • 2 slices whole-wheat bread
   • spread composed of 1 teaspoon softened sweet butter/marga-
     rine blend, mixed with ½ teaspoon prepared Dijon mustard
 1 medium banana
 1 cup skim milk

DINNER

½ Cornish hen (skinned), roasted
 1 cup cooked orzo (rice-shaped pasta) with homemade tomato
   sauce, sprinkled with:
   • minced fresh herbs
   • ½ teaspoon freshly grated Parmesan cheese
½ cup steamed green beans
¾ cup endive "coleslaw" prepared with:
   • ½ cup thinly sliced endive
   • ¼ cup shredded carrot
   • 1 tablespoon minced onion or scallion

- dash each salt and pepper
- 1 tablespoon oil and vinegar dressing, mixed with 2 table-spoons buttermilk

1 fresh peach or pear, *or* ¼ cup raisin-nut mix
1 cup skim milk

Snacks
(especially for kids at midafternoon)

• —————————————— •

If some of these snacks sound like junk foods, they are. But they're not. . . . They're healthful junk-food clones.

Some of these require no recipes. For those that do, refer to the recipe number in parentheses following the name of the snack, except for Fruit Butter, which has a page reference. Numbered recipes begin on page 183.

Fresh fruit

Fresh vegetables, cut up

Dried fruit, without preservatives

Popcorn, plain

Popcorn (9)

Raisin-nut mix

Crunchy Candy Balls (28)

Brown Sugar Cookies (26)

Fruit Butter (page 178)

Choc-O-Chip Ice Milk (95)

Soups (7, 33, 62, 78)

Jiffy Blueberry Jam (59)

Granola, commercial, without sugar or preservatives

Granola (1 and 1A)

Milk shakes (52, 74)

Chewy Brownies (32)

Stuffed Prunes (60)

Frozen Yogurt Tutti-Fruiti (61)

Fruit butters, commercial, without sugar or preservatives

Oatmeal Cookies (27)

Plain rice crackers, spread with commercial unsweetened jam

Peanut butter

Peanut butter with plain yogurt

• CHAPTER •

13

BREAKING YOUR FAMILY'S JUNK-FOOD HABIT

Healthful "Junk-Food" Clones

This may be the most important chapter in this book. If you and your husband can break the junk-food habit, you have a better chance for a healthful life. If your kids can break the junk-food habit, they have a better chance for a healthful life, *and* for a brighter life.

Yet it's not easy. The junk-food habit is an all-American habit. It's as natural to us as eating in and eating out. Almost all supermarket food is junk food—read the labels. All fast-food and take-out food, even the sophisticated kind, are junk foods, although there are no labels to read. If there were, *The New York Times* commented editorially in 1986, "the result might be a healthy change in the nation's eating habits."

But labeling and cautionary advice have not made any dents in megabillion-dollar supermarket junk-food sales, and won't in the newer but already $47 billion, and growing explosively, fast-food/take-out industry. When the plates are down, it's taste that counts —and, you can't get away from it, junk food tastes finger-lickin' good.

So what we're giving you and your kids to help start breaking the junk-food habit is healthful food that tastes like—and sometimes even looks like—junk food. Just imagine—

> *Healthful:*
> Whamburgers. Hamburger Buns. French Fries. Barbecue Ketchup. Bread and Butter Pickles. Copycat Chicken McNuggets.

Healthful:
Wonder-Ful Bread. Cuppa-Soup. Real Mayonnaise.
Canned-type Tomato and Chicken Soups.

Healthful:
Lasagna. TV Fish Dinner. Pizza. Tangy potato toppings.
Rich sauces. "Fried" Chicken.

Healthful:
Ice Creams—three flavor choices. Muffins—a half dozen
varieties. Brown Sugar Cookies. Crunchy Candy Balls.
Oatmeal Cookies. Apple Cake.

Healthful:
Popsicles. Jell-Os. Chewy Fruit Granola Bars. Fruit Butter.
Ice cream shakes. Popcorn. And even a—

Healthful:
Happy Birthday Cake!

How to Use Your Healthful "Junk-Food" Clones

It's simplicity itself. If you wish to replace a breakfast dish with a
healthful "junk food," just look under *Breakfast* in the list of clones
that follows, and substitute any for a matching dish in the Basic All-
Family Menu Plan. Do the same for *Lunch* and *Dinner*. "Matching"
means appetizer for appetizer, entree for entree, dessert for dessert,
and so forth.

Examples: For breakfast, instead of shredded wheat, why not a
healthful "junk-food" Chewy Fruit Granola Bar? For lunch, instead
of vegetable/egg–stuffed pita, how about a healthful "junk-food"
Whamburger on a Hamburger Bun? For dinner, instead of broiled
salmon, wouldn't you like a healthful "junk-food" TV Fish Dinner?

The **numbers in the parentheses** following each listed healthful
"junk-food" clone corresponds to the numbered recipes starting on
page 183. Some of them are so simple you can teach your kids to
make them. They're marked with a **K** for Kids.

There are two kinds of clones. One tastes more like real junk food than the other. (That's because some contain minute amounts of sugar, and some contain more fat than we ordinarily use.) These clones—still healthful by any standards—act as transitions (in-betweens) between real junk foods and our no-sugar, really low-fat clones.

Here's the trick: Use the in-between clones first. Then, when your kids get used to them—it's easy, because they do resemble junk foods—introduce the no-sugar, really low-fat clones. The tastes are so close to the in-betweens that your kids will get used to *them* fast. As a matter of fact, after a while your kids won't be able to tell the difference between the in-betweens and the real clones.

Then you can do one of two things:

You can drop the in-between clones from your menus, which is a shame because they're so tasty. Or you can follow our suggestions at the end of each in-between "junk-food" recipe, and convert it into a no-sugar, really low-fat "junk-food" clone. The recipes that can be converted are marked by an **asterisk (*) preceding the title.** Those **unasterisked** are already no-sugar, really low-fat "junk-food" clones.

All no-sugar, low-fat "junk-food" clones—those that don't need conversion and those that you convert—can be welcome additions to the Basic All-Family Menu Plan, permanently. Of course, you and your husband will make the same transition as your kids— from real junk foods to in-betweens to real "junk-food" clones. The whole family will break the junk-food habit together.

Healthful "Junk-Food" Clones

FOR BREAKFAST

*Granola, The Cereal (1)
*Granola, The Cereal and
    Snack (1A)
Chewy Fruit Granola Bars (2)
K   Tasty Muffins and
    Variations (3)

Wonder-Ful Bread (4)
*Breakfast Sausages (5)
K   Pancakes and Variations (6)

FOR LUNCH

Cuppa-Soup (7)

*"Canned" Cucumber-
  Zucchini Soup (8)

K   Popcorn (for soups or
      snacks) (9)

K   *Whamburger (10)

*Mushroom Pizza (11)

K   *Pizza Sauce (12)

*Spaghetti Sauce (13)

Fish and Shrimp Sticks (14)

*Creamed Mushrooms (15)

K   French Fries (16)

*Potato Salad (17)

K   *Bread and Butter Pickles (18)

K   Ketchup De-Lite (19)

Barbecue Ketchup (20)

*Real Mayonnaise (21)

K   Salad Dressing (22)

K   *Cheese Butter (23)

Hamburger Buns (24)

K   Applesauce (25)

*Brown Sugar Cookies (26)

K   *Oatmeal Cookies (27)

K   *Crunchy Candy Balls (28)

K   *3-Juice Jell-O or Popsicles (29)

*Peach Ice Cream (30)

*Black Cherry–Banana Ice
  Cream (31)

Chewy Brownies (32)

FOR DINNER

*"Canned" Tomato Soup (33)

Three TV Dinners (34)

Fish Dinner (34A)

*Crispy Fish Fillets

K   *Creamy Mashed Potatoes

K   Colorful Mixed Vegetables

Chicken Dinner (34B)

Chicken with Peppers

K   Brown Rice with
      Mushrooms

K   Steamed Peas

Mexican Dinner (34C)

Mexican Meatballs

K   Pinto Beans

K   Crunchy Broccoli

Super Salsa

*Copycat Chicken
  McNuggets (35)

K   *"Fried" Chicken (36)

*Chicken with Cheese (37)

Meat Loaf "Muffins" (38)

K   *Lasagna (39)

K   Rice Mix (40)

K   Top-of-the-Stove Stuffing
      (41)

K   *"Pouch-Type" Broccoli in
      Orange Sauce (42)

K   *Barbecue Sauce (43)

*Vegetable Slaw (44)

*Cranapple Sauce (45)

*Dessert Topping (46)

*Happy Birthday Cake (47)

*Plum Cake and Apple Cake
  (48)

*Blueberry Mousse (49)

"Supermarket" Cake (50)

Iced Banana Popsicles (51)

K   Ice Cream Milk Shake (52)

14

BRIGHT FOOD CAN BE GREAT FOOD

The New Four-Star Bright Cuisine

As great chefs over the last several years have interpreted the scientific findings of the "new nutrition" in their kitchens, millions of Americans have discovered that healthful cooking can be great cooking. Our new four-star Bright Cuisine is cooking in that tradition.

Catering to the palate, with the health of the whole family and particularly children's mental health in mind, our Bright Cuisine provides sweetness without sugar, creaminess without cream, tanginess without more than the right amount of salt, and tastiness without chemicals. It does this with selections mainly from the 265 Best Foods for Kids' Brains, and with none from the 181 Worst Foods for Kids' Brains.

Use our Bright Cuisine recipes as you use our healthful junk-food clones to add more excitement to The Basic All-Family Menu Plan. The list of Bright Cuisine recipes that follows is arranged according to *Breakfast, Lunch,* and *Dinner* dishes. Choose selections from them to replace similar dishes on the Basic Menus.

Make these savory superswaps, for example: At breakfast, swap hot oatmeal for Apple Pancakes with Blueberry Sauce. At lunch, swap low-sodium tomato juice for Broccoli Bisque. At dinner, swap a baked scrod or flounder for Shrimp with Banana.

But simple as these recipes are to make—every step is spelled out for you; and some are lettered **K,** which stands for even easy for kids to make (under your supervision)—some *do* take time.

Try to find the time. Start with just one of these superdelicious recipes a week. Then two. Then three. Soon you'll find cooking our way so much fun, and you'll enjoy the plaudits of your family so much, you'll want to cook more and more.

Dishes of the Bright Cuisine

The **numbers in parentheses** following each title correspond to the numbered recipes starting on page 183.

FOR BREAKFAST

Whole-Wheat Bread (53)

No-Knead Raisin Bread (54)

K   Whole-Wheat Popovers (55)

K   Bacon-Tasting Onions and Eggs (56)

Apple Pancake (57)

Blueberry Sauce (58)

Jiffy Blueberry Jam (59)

K   Stuffed Prunes (60)

K   Frozen Yogurt Tutti-Fruiti (61)

FOR LUNCH

Broccoli Bisque (62)

Tofu Casserole—It's a Whole Meal! (63)

K   Veal Burgers (64)

Barbecued Swordfish (65)

Chinese-Style Sautéed Shrimp (66)

K   Versatile Sardine Salad (67)

Roast Turkey Thighs (68)

Ginger Chicken (69)

Pasta and Beans (70)

K   Broccoli-Chicken Salad (71)

K   Colorful Salad with Fruit Dressing (72)

Sautéed Apples and Zucchini (73)

K   Peanut Butter Milk Shake (74)

Applesauce Pudding Squares (75)

K   Apple Sauté (76)

Beige Ice Cream (77)

FOR DINNER

New-Fashioned Mushroom and Barley Soup (78)

Three Marinades (79)

Barbecue Marinade (79A)

Indian-Style Marinade (79B)

Cranberry Spice Marinade (79C)

Chicken with Apples (80)

Poached Chicken with Creamy Sauce (81)

Roast Chicken with Rosy Sauce (82)

Stewed Chicken with Apricots (83)

Scallop of Veal (84)

Braised Veal (85)

Lamb Patties (86)

Mixed Meat Stew (87)

Shrimp with Banana (88)

Fillet of Sole in Fruit Sauce (89)

New Coleslaw (90)

Corn and Peppers (91)

Fast and Simple Kasha
   (Buckwheat Groats) (92)

Potato Pancakes (93)

Eggplant Caviar (94)

Choc-O-Chip Ice Milk (95)

15

PREGNANCY, BREASTFEEDING,
THE BRAIN'S SECOND BIRTH

Adapting the Basic All-Family Menu Plan to Your Kids' and Your Special Needs

The two tables on the following pages make it simple to adapt the Basic All-Family Menu Plan to your requirements during pregnancy and breastfeeding, and to your child's requirements during the brain's second birth, from age 1 to age 5—in accordance with the Mother's Milk Principle. For guidelines on your kids' diet from 4 months to age 1, see pages 112–16.

The tables are based on the path-breaking achievements of Alice White, the noted nutritionist, and of Dorcas Demasio, who formulated brilliantly imaginative Mother's Milk Principle diets for Dr. Ralph Minear.

Adapting the Menus to Pregnancy and Breastfeeding

1. Look over your daily menu and identify each dish by its Food Group. To make the identifications, refer to the 265 Best Foods for Your Kids' Brains (pages 126–33), which are arranged according to Food Groups. Veal, for example, is in the ANIMAL FOODS/ EGGS Food Group.
2. Locate the Food Group on Table 1 (opposite). Go to the "Nonpregnant" column and subtract the number you find there from the corresponding number in the "Pregnant" column. The difference is the additional serving to include in your meal.

Table 1. **ADAPTING THE BASIC ALL-FAMILY MENU PLAN FOR PREGNANCY AND BREASTFEEDING**

Food Group	Serving Size	Number of Servings		
		Nonpregnant	Pregnant	Breastfeeding
1. ANIMAL FOODS/EGGS	Meat, 4 ounces, cooked	1	1½	2
	Eggs, 3 large	*	*	*
2. MILK/YOGURT/CHEESE†	Milk/yogurt, 1 cup	2†	4‡	5‡
	Cheese, 1 ounce			
3. GRAINS	1 cup, cooked	2	2	2
4. BREADS/CRACKERS/INGREDIENTS	Bread, 1 slice	2	3	3
	Rolls, ½ roll			
	Crackers			
5. LEGUMES/NUTS/SEEDS	1 cup, cooked	1	1	1
	1 square, tofu			
6. VITAMIN-C FRUITS/VEGETABLES	¾ to 1 cup	1	2	2
	same for juices			
7. DARK GREEN VEGETABLES	¾ to 1 cup	1	1	2
	same for juices			
8. OTHER FRUITS/VEGETABLES	¾ to 1 cup	1	1	2
	same for juices			
9. FATS	1 tablespoon	1	2	2
10. SWEETS	Small quantities	—	—	—
11. HERBS/SPICES/CONDIMENTS/ FLAVORINGS	Small quantities	—	—	—

* No more than three a week. Count one egg as ⅓ serving.
† Skim or nonfat; plain low-fat yogurt.
‡ Whole milk; regular yogurt.

NOTE: "Contrary to previous theory," Boston Children's Hospital reports, "recent studies have shown that pregnant women may need additional salt. . . . Two to 3 grams of sodium are recommended because the normal fluid retention somewhat increases the body's sodium needs." You can obtain the recommended amount by adding a little less than 1 to 1½ teaspoons of salt to *your* food daily.

Example: Veal is 1 in the "Nonpregnant" column and 1½ in the "Pregnant" column. The difference is ½ serving, which should be added to your dish. For basic serving size, see under the column headed "Serving Size."

3. Repeat this simple process when you're breastfeeding by sub-tracting the number in the "Nonpregnant" column from the number in the "Breastfeeding" column.

Adapting the Menus to Kids Ages 1 Through 5

1. Identify each dish by its Food Group, a you did in step 1 for adapting the menus to pregnancy and breastfeeding.
2. Locate the Food Group on Table 2 (opposite). The number under the column corresponding to your child's age represents the number of servings to feed your child.

Example: The dish is veal, and your child is age 3½. The Food Group is ANIMAL FOODS/EGGS and the number under "Age 3 to 4" is 2½. You'll feed your child bright with that number of serv-ings. Basic serving sizes for children under 5 are, of course, less than for adults. You'll find them in the "Serving Size" column.

When your kids reach age 5, you face a choice: You can feed them on the low-fat Basic All-Family Menu Plan, or you can continue to feed them until about age 12 on whole milk and whole-milk prod-ucts.

Argument for the low-fat diet is that it's a defense against heart attack and other degenerative diseases. Argument for the higher-fat diet is that your kids' brains continue to grow in size to adolescence, with significant increases in the vital "pathways in the brain," a growth requiring a greater fat intake than adults'. On a fully supple-mented diet, this pro-higher-fat argument continues, the threat of heart attack is likely to be defused.

The decision is yours to arrive at in consultation with a doctor well qualified in nutrition—and that's the way all decisions should be made concerning the nutritional welfare of yourself, and of your child, from preconception to the threshold of adolescence.

Table 2. **ADAPTING THE BASIC ALL-FAMILY MENU PLAN FOR KIDS AGES 1 to 5**

Food Group	Serving Size	Age:	Number of Servings			
			1 to 2	2 to 3	3 to 4	4 to 5
1. ANIMAL FOODS/EGGS	Meat, 1 ounce		2	2½	2½	3
	1 egg					
2. MILK/YOGURT/CHEESE	Milk/yogurt, ½ cup		6	7	8	8
	Cheese, ½ ounce					
3. GRAINS	¼ cup, cooked		1	1	1½	1½
4. BREAD/CRACKERS/INGREDIENTS	Bread, ½ slice		5	6	6½	7
	2 wheat crackers					
	1 graham cracker					
5. LEGUMES/NUTS/SEEDS	½ cup, cooked		1	1	1½	1½
6. VITAMIN-C FRUITS/VEGETABLES	Fruits, ½ cup		1	1	1½	1½
	Vegetables, 3 tablespoons					
	Juices, ½ cup					
7. DARK GREEN VEGETABLES	3 tablespoons		1	1	1½	1½
8. OTHER FRUITS/VEGETABLES	½ cup		4	5	5	6
9. FATS	1 teaspoon		3–3½	3½	4–4½	4–4½
10. SWEETS	Small quantities		—	—	—	—
11. HERBS/SPICES/CONDIMENTS/ FLAVORINGS	Small quantities		—	—	—	—

159

• CHAPTER •
16

VITAMINS AND MINERALS

The Bright Supplements for You and Your Kids

Processing, even of fresh foods, has so diminished our foods' natural supply of vitamins and minerals that even the best possible diet of American food must be supplemented to reach optimal health levels for body and mind. The supplement formulas recommended in the following pages are available by mail from NutriGuard Research, P.O. Box 865, Encinitas, California 92024. We have no financial interest of any kind in that company; and the selection of the formulas was made on the basis of merit alone.

RDAs are Recommended Dietary Allowances set by the Food and Nutrition Board, National Academy of Sciences–National Research Council to prevent the onset of vitamin/mineral–deprivation diseases. ODAs are Optimal Dietary Allowances, on the whole higher than RDAs, established by some medical nutrition scientists as necessary to help prevent preclinical symptoms of those diseases. All the supplements recommended—for preconception, for pregnancy and breastfeeding, and for kids from ages 2 to 12—are ODA formulations.

These are not "megadoses," extraordinary large quantities of vitamins/minerals, even though the therapeutic uses of megadoses have been helpful in treating many kinds of children's mental diseases.

Dr. Bernard Rimland has documented successes with numerous cases of autism (a disease that prevents a child from relating or communicating meaningfully with other human beings). Dr. Abram Hoffer, a Canadian Public Health Department official, and Dr. Henry Osmond, a New Jersey neuropsychiatric specialist, have improved the condition of schizophrenics (victims of a disease characterized by delusions, hallucinations and loss of a sense of reality). Dr. Henry Turkel, a Michigan pediatrician specializing in retarded children, has reported significant reversals of retardation, even among children born with Down's disease (mongolism). Dr. Allan Cott has recorded major victories over a wide range of learning disabilities.

But megadoses must be prescribed and closely monitored by physicians with in-depth backgrounds in nutrition. Megadoses of vitamins/minerals could, for some children, be dangerous and even fatal.

Dr. Earl L. Mindell, a leader in establishing safe and sensible levels of vitamin/mineral supplementation for mother and child, says, "I firmly believe [they] are as important as love . . . for the continuing vitality and happiness of your children in the years ahead."

A Non-Pregnancy ODA Supplement

•

This formulation belongs to a category of multi-vitamin/mineral combinations called "insurance formulas." "An insurance formula," writes one of the nation's leading experts on commercial nutrient supplements, Dr. Sheldon Hendler, "is one that contains at least the RDAs as well as upper limits of safe and adequate doses of all essential trace minerals, major minerals, and vitamins. Insurance formulas, at their best, strive for a balance of nutrients that seem optimal given present knowledge. They are designed to help prevent the premature onset of degenerative diseases."

Dr. Hendler adds, "I have found only two insurance formulas that I can recommend." The superior of these two products, judging from Dr. Hendler's analysis, is called Broad Spectrum. Information for the tabular form is provided here. Manufacturer's recommended dose is 3 tablets with breakfast and 3 with dinner. Broad Spectrum is also available as a flavored powder.

6 tablets supply

A (as Beta Carotene)	25,000	IU
(as Retinyl Palmitate)	5,000	IU
B₁ (Thiamine HCl)	10	mg
B₂ (Riboflavin)	10	mg
Niacinamide	100	mg
Calcium Pantothenate	50	mg
B₆ (Pyrodoxine HCl)	50	mg
B₁₂ (Cobalamin Concentrate)	30	mcg
Folic Acid	400	mcg
Biotin	100	mcg
C (Ascorbic Acid)	1,000	mg
D₃ (Cholecalciferol)	400	IU
E (d-alpha-Tocopheryl Acetate)	400	IU
K₁ (Phytonadione)	100	mcg

6 tablets supply

Choline (Bitartrate)	250	mg
Calcium (Carbonate)	1,000	mg
Magnesium (Oxide)	400	mg
Zinc (Gluconate)	30	mg
Iron (Ferrous Fumarate)	18	mg
Manganese (Gluconate)	10	mg
Copper (Gluconate)	3	mg
Selenium (Nutrition 21 Yeast)	200	mcg
Chromium (Nutrition 21 Yeast)	100	mcg
(as Chromium Acetate)	100	mcg
Iodine (Potassium Iodide)	150	mcg
Molybdenum (Sodium Molybdate)	150	mcg
Magnesium (Magnesium Trisilicate)	20	mg

NOTE: IU stands for International Units; mg for milligrams; mcg for micrograms.

162

A Pregnancy and Breastfeeding ODA Supplement

•

This insurance formula is the only one we know that provides at least pregnancy RDAs for all vitamins and minerals (except phosphorus, which is adequately supplied by our All-Family Menu Plan). Called Pre-Natal Formula, it contains ample amounts of iron, folic acid and calcium, vital for the health of mother and child during the crucial months of child bearing and breastfeeding. For optimal safety, beta carotene is the vitamin A source. Manufacturer's recommended dose is 3 tablets with breakfast and 3 with dinner.

	6 tablets supply
A (Beta Carotene)	10,000 IU
B₁ (Thiamine HCI)	3.4 mg
B₂ (Riboflavin)	4 mg
Niacinamide	40 mg
Calcium Pantothenate	20 mg
B₆ (Pyrodoxine HCl)	5 mg
B₁₂ (Cobalamin Concentrate)	16 mcg
Biotin	300 mcg
Folic Acid	800 mcg
C (Ascorbic Acid)	240 mg
D₃ (Cholecalciferol)	600 IU
E (d-alpha-Tocopheryl Acetate)	60 IU

	6 tablets supply
K₁ (Phytonadione)	100 mcg
Calcium (Carbonate)	1,300 mg
Magnesium (Oxide)	450 mg
Iron (Ferrous Fumarate)	50 mg
Zinc (Gluconate)	25 mg
Manganese (Gluconate)	5 mg
Copper (Gluconate)	2 mg
Selenium (L-Selenomethionine)	200 mcg
Chromium (Chromium Acetate)	200 mcg
Molybdenum (Sodium Molybdate)	150 mcg
Silicon (Magnesium Trisilicate)	20 mg

NOTE: IU stands for International Units; mg for milligrams; mcg for micrograms.

163

An ODA Supplement for Your Kids

• —————————————— •

There are no specific numerical recommendations for supplementation between birth and age 2. An iron supplement is usually added to baby formulas and foods to meet the RDA, but supplementation is at the discretion of your nutritionally knowledgeable doctor. Dr. Lendon Smith, the renowned pediatrician, prescribes an early start to supplementation with "brewer's yeast and wheat germ [excellent sources of B-complex vitamins] mixed in old-fashioned peanut butter . . . and vitamin C as a concentrated powder." But he's vague as to when to start and how much to give.

That's as it should be. Kids between birth and age 2 change so rapidly, and their needs are so individual, that no general supplementation formula is applicable. Consult your nutrition-trained and -experienced physician.

This insurance formula for children, sold under the name Child's Chewable, is the only one we know containing selenium and chromium. Selenium not only fortifies your child's immune system and fights cancer, but is also an essential ingredient of glutathione peroxidase, a biochemical manufactured in your child's body that several studies have linked to I.Q. Chromium plays a vital role in the metabolism of glucose, the energy source for your child's brain.

This product contains no milk, wheat, yeast or soy protein, which may produce allergic reactions in some children. It is also free of artificial flavors, colorings and preservatives. For optimal safety it contains iron in its elemental form and vitamin A as beta-carotene. Phosphorus and calcium, which do not appear in the formula, are adequately supplied by our All-Family Menu Plan adapted for kids. Manufacturer's recommended dose is 1 to 2 wafers a day. The wafers are fruit flavored.

	2 wafers supply	
A (Beta Carotene)	10,000	IU
B_1 (Thiamine HCl)	1.5	mg
B_2 (Riboflavin)	1.7	mg
Niacinamide	20	mg
Calcium Pantothenate	10	mg
B_6 (Pyrodoxine HCl)	2	mg
B_{12} (Cobalamin Concentrate)	6	mcg
Folic Acid	400	mcg
Biotin	100	mcg
C (Ascorbic Acid)	240	mg
D_1 (Cholecalciferol)	200	IU
E (d-alpha-Tocopherol Acetate)	30	IU
K_1 (Phytonadione)	100	mcg
Magnesium (Chelate)	80	mg
Zinc (Chelate)	10	mg
Iron (Micronized Elemental)	18	mg
Manganese (Chelate)	5	mg
Copper (Chelate)	2	mg
Selenium (L-Selenomethionine)	150	mcg
Chromium (Chromium Acetate)	150	mcg
Iodine (Potassium Iodide)	150	mcg
Molybdenum (sodium Molybdate)	150	mcg

NOTE: IU stands for International Units; mg for milligrams; mcg for micrograms.

The Magic of Cooking Bright

Before You Begin

We were in a supermarket in Tampa, Florida (food shops are our first destination wherever we go), and a woman wheeling a cart packed higher than the rim with frozen TV dinners, ice creams, sugared breakfast cereals, and packages on packages of cakes and candies, stopped us and said:

"Saw you on TV, and let me tell you something. Nutrition is no good if it don't taste good."

She's right.

And that's what scientists, doctors, and nutritionists who tell you what you should eat forget. You *can't* eat it if it "don't taste good." And neither can your kids.

The magic of cooking bright *makes* it taste good, makes healthful but dull, blah, *ugh*-ly ingredients taste not just good, but great— and that's why it's magic. It's a magic that can be learned, and this cookbook shows you how.

If you haven't cooked before—*really* cooked—you have one of life's greatest experiences before you. It opens a world of infinite delights. Cooking is a creative joy that can turn anyone into an artist. Share that joy with your husband and your kids. For your spouse, as it is for you, it's a new adventure in living. For your kids, it's that, and an exciting stimulant to the growth of new neurotransmitter pathways of learning in the brain. For your whole family, there's no more satisfying experience than eating together the food you've cooked together.

To put the magical taste into your dishes, begin by stocking up on those ingredients that are pure sorcery in the kitchen—herbs and spices (you'll find them listed under Food Group 11, page 132). But that's just the start of your cooking wizardry. As you learn by doing, recipe by recipe, you'll concoct marvels of marinades with them, and sautéed delights that can add excitement to your menus.

Shopping for the ingredients in these recipes is easy, because you can find almost everything in your supermarket, including the herbs and spices, which are growing more popular every day. But there are a few items more readily available in health-food stores than elsewhere and here they are (including some for in-between "junk-food" clones only):

Black cherry concentrate; blackstrap molasses, third extraction; baking powder (double action), without aluminum; buckwheat flour; carob powder and chips, unsweetened; coconut, unsweetened; cold pressed oils; date powder (sometimes called date sugar); dried dates and apricots without preservatives; grain coffee; honey, uncooked, unfiltered; low-sodium vegetable seasoning; plain whole-milk yogurt; sesame seeds, unhulled; smoked yeast (sometimes called bacon yeast); wheat flakes; whole kasha (buckwheat groats); and whole-wheat pastry flour. If you need specific sources for ingredients, write to Francine Prince care of the publisher.

And some healthful hints:

When no specific oil is mentioned in a recipe, select any from Food Group 9, page 131. They're all among the most healthful.

Be sure to remove the skin from your poultry. More than 20 percent of the chicken's fat—it's saturated to boot—lurks under the skin.

Don't use the skins of vegetables unless they're well scrubbed to help rid them of harmful additives. In Cooking Bright recipes, onions, shallots, garlic, fresh ginger, and turnip are peeled; carrots are peeled or well-scrubbed; and zucchini is well-scrubbed but not peeled.

Wash and dry all meats, fish, chicken, vegetables, and fruit *always*. That helps get rid of some of the dangerous chemical additives, and some of the pathogenic bacteria. (One out of three chickens can infect you and your kids with botulism.) After cutting, washing, and drying any food, thoroughly wash your hands, your cutting board, and any utensil touched by the food.

If you're using Cooking Bright recipes as a basis for baby foods for your under-1-year-old, eliminate honey and replace with concentrated fruit juice.

Don't use copper or aluminum cookware. They're anti-vitamin. Iron pots are fine, though; they release much-needed iron into your food. Nonstick skillets cut the need for fat; so use them, too.

To preserve the vitamin content in fruits and vegetables, steam (or cook in as little water as possible), don't prepare them far ahead of cooking time, and don't let them soak too long in water (except dried beans and other legumes). Save your vitamin-rich cooking water for soups and broths.

And some cooking tips:

Depending on the type of skillet used (enameled, cast iron, nonstick), cooking times and liquid remaining will differ. Cast-iron skillets, which conduct heat rapidly and retain heat, will brown foods and cook them more rapidly than nonstick or enameled skillets.

Should you run out of My Chicken Broth, or want to extend the broth you have on hand, use 1 teaspoon low-sodium vegetable seasoning per 1 cup boiling water. Taste will differ, but you'll like it.

It's not inconsistent to start with no-salt-added canned tomatoes and tomato juice, then add some salt. Here's why: Most canned salt-added tomato products contribute 250 to 500 or more milligrams (mg.) sodium per serving. Adding just ⅛ to ¼ teaspoon salt to a no-salt-added canned tomato or tomato juice recipe serving four boosts sodium per serving by only about 90 to 180 mg., amounts more healthful for children and adults as well.

I use large eggs in all recipes calling for eggs.

To get the most out of Cooking Bright bread recipes, keep this in mind: The amount of flour is approximate because there is a wide variation in the ability of flour to absorb moisture. Should a recipe call for 3½ to 4 cups, always start with the lesser amount. You can always *add* more flour but you can't *remove* what you've already put in. Too much flour will produce a dense, hard, untasty loaf. Rising time will vary depending upon humidity and air temperatures in *your* kitchen. Baking times vary slightly with the efficiency of *your* oven.

In Cooking Bright recipes, milk means *whole* milk and plain yogurt means plain *whole* yogurt. Use the skim or low-fat varieties only when specified. No substitutions, please, for health and culinary reasons.

The Cooking Bright recipes that follow are Francine Prince originals. For the remainder of "The Magic of Cooking Bright" she will be guiding you in their use as if she were giving you personal lessons.

Now enter the magic world of cooking bright. . . .

The Magic Mixers: Recipes to Make All Recipes Taste Better

Following are ten mixers that could change your life in the kitchen. They're your gateway to expedience, flavor, and economy; and they're so versatile, you'll discover many exciting new ways to use them.

I've included measurements for sample-size portions (enough for at least one recipe) of my dry mixers and My Frozen Vegetable Mix so you can try them, if you like, before making up large batches.

Since developing these mixers, I've found I'm utterly lost without them. I store them on my shelf or in my freezer or refrigerator at all times for whipping up quick batches of muffins, cakes, pancakes, spaghetti sauce, seasoned popcorn, and many other of our favorites.

For the recipes I use them in, see USED IN THESE RECIPES at the bottom of each Magic Mix recipe. The numbers in parentheses refer to the numbers of those recipes. Recipes are arranged numerically beginning on page 183.

Since my Magic Mixers significantly speed up the preparation of so many delightful-tasting dishes (you can cut preparation time by at least 50 percent), you'll find it easy to prepare healthful and exciting dishes for your family every day.

MY MUFFIN AND CAKE MIX

For about 2½ cups	For about 15½ cups	
1½ cups	9 cups	unbleached flour
½ cup	3 cups	whole-wheat pastry flour
2½ teaspoons	5 tablespoons	baking powder
2 tablespoons	¾ cup	nonfat dry milk solids
⅛ teaspoon	¾ teaspoon	salt
½ teaspoon	3 teaspoons	ground cinnamon
2 tablespoons	¾ cup	sugar
2 tablespoons	¾ cup	tightly packed date powder
2 tablespoons	¾ cup	regular wheat germ

1. Into an 8- or 9-quart pot or bowl, sift flours, baking powder, milk, salt, and cinnamon. Add sugar, date powder, and wheat germ. With 2 large spoons, stir continually, turning over mixture many times, until well mixed.
2. To store, spoon into labeled containers, leaving 2 inches from top. Before measuring, stir mixture (do not shake), turning over ingredients several times. Then spoon into measuring cups.

NOTE: This recipe may be prepared without sugar. For about 2½ cups, eliminate sugar, increase date powder measurement to ¼ cup, and cinnamon measurement to ¾ teaspoon. For about 15½ cups, eliminate sugar, increase date powder measurement to 1½ cups, and cinnamon measurement to 3½ teaspoons.

USED IN THESE RECIPES:

   Tasty Muffins and Variations (3)
   Brown Sugar Cookies (26)
   Happy Birthday Cake (47)
   Plum Cake and Apple Cake (48)
   Applesauce Pudding Squares (75)

MY FROZEN VEGETABLE MIX

For about 3 tightly packed cups	*For about 9 tightly packed cups*	
2	6	*medium carrots, peeled*
2	6	*medium onions, peeled*
1	3	*medium sweet green pepper(s), seeded*
2	6	*large ribs celery, ends trimmed*
3	9	*large cloves garlic, peeled*
1	3	*½-inch slice(s), fresh ginger, peeled*
½ cup	1½ cups	*firmly packed parsley florets*

1. Cut carrots, onions, green pepper, and celery into 2-inch pieces. If outer stalks of pascal celery are used, peel back or cut away coarse strings. Cut each clove garlic in half, and ginger into quarters. Fit food processor with steel blade. Arrange cut vegetables in layers, starting with carrots and ginger, then adding layers of celery, parsley, onion, garlic, and green pepper. Coarse-chop by processing on/off 4 to 6 times. (If 9 cups are being prepared, process in 3 batches.)

2. Transfer to several ½-cup and 1-cup plastic bags or freezerproof containers. Close tightly and freeze.
3. When ready to use, let stand at room temperature for 15 minutes. Break up. Mixture is now ready to use. Complete defrosting is not necessary.

USED IN THESE RECIPES:

My "Canned" Chicken Broth (page 178)
Cuppa-Soup (7)
"Canned" Cucumber-Zucchini Soup (8)
Pizza Sauce (12)
Meat Loaf "Muffins" (38)
Cranapple Sauce (45)
New-Fashioned Mushroom and Barley Soup (78)
Chicken with Apples (80)
Braised Veal (85)
Mixed Meat Stew (87)

MY PANCAKE MIX

For about 1⅔ cups	For about 10½ cups	
1¼ cups	7½ cups	unbleached flour
2 tablespoons	¾ cup	stone-ground whole-wheat flour
1 tablespoon	6 tablespoons	regular wheat germ
1½ teaspoons	3 tablespoons	baking powder
¼ teaspoon	1½ teaspoons	ground cinnamon
⅛ teaspoon	¾ teaspoon	salt
1 tablespoon	6 tablespoons	date powder
¼ cup	1½ cups	nonfat dry milk solids

1. Into an 8- or 9-quart pot or bowl, combine all ingredients. With 2 large spoons, stir continually, turning over mixture many times, until well mixed.
2. To store, spoon into labeled containers, leaving 2 inches from top. Before measuring, stir mixture (do not shake), turning over ingredients several times. Then spoon into measuring cups.

USED IN THESE RECIPES:

Pancakes and Variations (6)
No-Knead Raisin Bread (54)
Apple Pancake (57)
Potato Pancakes (93)

MY SHAKE AND BAKE-ALIKE

For about 2 cups	*For about 6⅓ cups*	
¼ cup	¾ cup	toasted unhulled sesame seeds
3 tablespoons	½ cup	regular wheat germ
½ cup	1½ cups	fine toasted bread crumbs
⅓ cup	1 cup	stone-ground yellow cornmeal
¼ cup	¾ cup	each stone-ground whole-wheat flour and unbleached flour
¼ cup	¾ cup	freshly grated Parmesan cheese
1 tablespoon	3 tablespoons	finely chopped lemon rind
1 teaspoon	1 tablespoon	ground ginger
½ teaspoon	1½ teaspoons	each dry mustard and ground cinnamon
5 teaspoons	¼ cup plus 1 tablespoon	onion powder
Pinch	¼ teaspoon	cayenne pepper
½ teaspoon	1½ teaspoons	salt

1. Into an 8- or 9-quart pot or bowl, combine all ingredients. With 2 large spoons, stir continually, turning over mixture many times, until well mixed.
2. To store, spoon into labeled containers, leaving 2 inches from top. Before measuring, stir mixture (do not shake), turning over ingredients several times. Then spoon into measuring cups.

USED IN THESE RECIPES:

Breakfast Sausages (5)
Whamburger (10)
Fish and Shrimp Sticks (14)
Crispy Fish Fillets (34A)
"Fried" Chicken (36)
Veal Burgers (64)
Lamb Patties (86)

MY SEASONING MIX

For a little less than 3 tablespoons	For a little less than ⅔ cup	
2 teaspoons	2 tablespoons	minced dried onion
1 teaspoon	1 tablespoon	minced dried garlic
1 tablespoon	3 tablespoons	low-sodium vegetable seasoning
1 teaspoon	1 tablespoon	smoked yeast (available in health-food stores)
½ teaspoon	1½ teaspoons	onion powder
¼ teaspoon	¾ teaspoon	salt
1 teaspoon	1 tablespoon	dried dillweed
½ teaspoon	1½ teaspoons	dried parsley flakes
¼ teaspoon	¾ teaspoon	ground cinnamon
½ teaspoon	1½ teaspoons	dried sage leaves

1. Combine all ingredients in a small bowl, gently stirring to blend. Transfer to jar. Store, tightly closed in cool dry place.
2. Because heavier ingredients tend to drift toward bottom of mix after standing a while, stir well before each use.

USED IN THESE RECIPES:

Popcorn (9)
Salad Dressing (22)
Top-of-the-Stove Stuffing (41)
New Coleslaw (90)

MY SPICY MIX

For about 2½ tablespoons	For a little less than ⅔ cup	
1½ teaspoons	2 tablespoons	onion powder
¾ teaspoon	1 tablespoon	dried parsley flakes
¾ teaspoon	1 tablespoon	dried rosemary leaves, crushed
1½ teaspoons	2 tablespoons	dried oregano leaves, crushed
¾ teaspoon	1 tablespoon	mild curry powder
½ teaspoon	2 teaspoons	ground ginger
¼ teaspoon	1 teaspoon	ground allspice
1½ teaspoons	2 tablespoons	chili con carne seasoning (see Note)
¼ teaspoon	1 teaspoon	salt
¼ teaspoon	1 teaspoon	ground cumin

1. Combine all ingredients in small bowl, gently stirring to blend. Transfer to jar. Store, tightly closed in cool dry place.
2. Because heavier ingredients tend to drift toward bottom of mix after standing a while, stir well before each use.

NOTE: Chili con carne "seasoning" contains no salt. Chili con carne "powder" contains an appreciable amount of salt. The "seasoning" has a milder flavor.

USED IN THESE RECIPES:

Breakfast Sausages (5)
Whamburger (10)
Creamed Mushrooms (15)
French Fries (16)
Potato Salad (17)
Salad Dressing (22)
Colorful Salad with Fruit Dressing (72)
Sautéed Apples and Zucchini (73)
New-Fashioned Mushroom and Barley Soup (78)
Barbecue Marinade (79A)
Chicken with Apples (80)
Roast Chicken with Rosy Sauce (82)
Stewed Chicken with Apricots (83)
Lamb Patties (86)
Mixed Meat Stew (87)
Fillet of Sole in Fruit Sauce (89)
Fast and Simple Kasha (Buckwheat Groats) (92)

MY FRUIT BUTTER—a sweetening staple

You don't have to sample this one; it's sweet-tooth proof.

8 ounces dried dates (without preservatives added)
8 ounces dried apricots (without preservatives added), well rinsed
1 cup tightly packed dark raisins

1 2-inch piece vanilla bean, split
2 cups unsweetened apple juice
1 teaspoon ground cinnamon
2 tablespoons frozen pineapple or orange juice concentrate

1. Place all ingredients in heavy-bottomed 1½- to 2-quart saucepan. Bring to boil. Reduce heat to simmering point. Cover and simmer for 20 minutes, stirring from time to time. Remove from heat and let stand, covered, until cooled. (Most of liquid will be absorbed.)
2. Using food mill, puree one-third of mixture at a time, reserving solids. Store in tightly closed glass container for up to 3 weeks.

YIELD: About 2½ cups puree; about 1 cup solids

SERVING SUGGESTIONS: Serve as an infant fruit puree; it has far more flavor and nutrition than any commercial fruit puree.

Serve puree or solids as breakfast food or dessert, plain, topped with ice-cold undiluted evaporated milk, or mixed with desired amount of plain yogurt.

USED IN THESE RECIPES:

Black Cherry–Banana Ice Cream (31)
Happy Birthday Cake (47)
Plum Cake and Apple Cake (48)
Blueberry Sauce (58)
Applesauce Pudding Squares (75)

MY "CANNED" CHICKEN BROTH

My Chicken Broth, a treasurehouse of nutrients and flavors, is used in many recipes. It's a lighter, quicker-cooking version of traditional chicken stock. Replete with flavorful essences of chicken, vegetables, and herbs, it does wonders for soups, sauces, and gravies. It's easy to make, simmering away happily by itself while you're busy with other chores.

1 *broiling chicken, including neck and gizzard, skinned and butterflied*
6 *cups water*
2 *medium onions, coarsely chopped*
2 *carrots, peeled and thickly sliced*
4 *large cloves garlic, coarsely chopped*
3 *ribs celery, cut into chunks*
6 *large sprigs parsley or dill or a combination of both*

1 *½-inch slice fresh ginger, peeled and chopped*
⅓ *cup peeled and diced white turnip*
¼ *pound fresh mushrooms, ends trimmed, rinsed, dried, and coarsely chopped*
½ *teaspoon each dried thyme and sage leaves*

1. Lay chicken, meaty side down, in large heavy kettle. Add balance of ingredients except thyme and sage. Bring slowly to gentle boil. Skim surface with large spoon. Add thyme and sage. Cover and simmer for 2 hours, stirring from time to time.
2. With slotted spoon remove chicken. (Reserve for sandwiches, salads, or main course, dressed with Creamed Mushrooms (page 196). Pour broth and solids into fine meshed strainer or chinois with large bowl underneath. Press out juices. Then strain through washed cotton cheesecloth.
3. Transfer to freezeproof containers. Cover tightly and refrigerate overnight. Discard fat that rises to top. Clear, virtually fat-free broth is ready to use.

YIELD: About 5½ cups

STORING SUGGESTIONS: For a child's meal, or as an addition to any recipe calling for chicken broth, for quick access to 2-tablespoon measures, fill each cube of large ice-cube trays with 2 tablespoons fat-skimmed broth; freeze. Remove cubes and store in double plastic bags for instant use.

NOTES: If you're stocked with My Frozen Vegetable Mix (page 173), substitute 2 cups of mix for onions, carrots, garlic, celery, parsley, and ginger. Continue with balance of recipe.

If you're preparing the recipe as written, vegetable chunks may be removed from the strainer before pressing out the juices in step 2, and reserved for a delicious meal for baby. Strain solids, or puree in a baby food grinder or food mill, or chop with knife. Broth or plain yogurt may be added to adjust the consistency. There should be about 1 cup puree, which can be frozen and used as needed.

USED IN THESE RECIPES:

Light Mayonnaise (this chapter)
Cuppa-Soup (7)
"Canned" Cucumber-Zucchini Soup (8)
Spaghetti Sauce (13)
Creamed Mushrooms (15)

Potato Salad (17)
Barbecue Ketchup (20)
"Canned" Tomato Soup (33)
Chicken with Peppers (34B)
Brown Rice with Mushrooms (34B)
Pinto Beans (optional) (34C)
Chicken with Cheese (37)
Meat Loaf "Muffins" (38)
Rice Mix (40)
Top-of-the-Stove Stuffing (optional) (41)
Broccoli Bisque (62)
Tofu Casserole (63)
Roast Turkey Thighs (68)
Pasta and Beans (70)
New-Fashioned Mushroom and Barley Soup (78)
Barbecue Marinade (79A)
Poached Chicken with Creamy Sauce (81)
Roast Chicken with Rosy Sauce (82)
Scallop of Veal (84)
Braised Veal (85)
Shrimp with Banana (88)
Fast and Simple Kasha (Buckwheat Groats) (92)

TWO KINDS OF MAYONNAISE

Successful, delicious mayonnaise, without sugar, excess salt, and preservatives, and with healthful oils, may be prepared several ways, but my favorite is: the electric mayonnaise maker way. It never fails; and thick, creamy mayonnaise is prepared effortlessly in 30 seconds. The two mayonnaises that follow transform the plainest foods into highly pleasing, luscious-tasting delights. Just a little goes a long way.

MY REAL MAYONNAISE

1 egg yolk	1/8 teaspoon cayenne pepper
1 teaspoon prepared Dijon mustard	1/2 cup each Italian olive oil and peanut
1/2 teaspoon fresh lemon juice	or corn oil
1/2 teaspoon white or apple cider vinegar	Black or white pepper, to taste
1/4 teaspoon salt	

To prepare by hand: Combine first 6 listed ingredients plus 1 tablespoon oil in bowl. Whisk until well blended. While whisking, slowly dribble in oil, a drop at a time, until half of oil is used. Then pour in a slow steady stream while whisking, until thickened. Taste. Sprinkle with additional lemon juice and pepper to taste, and whisk again.

To prepare with food processor: Fit processor with steel blade. Combine first 6 listed ingredients and 1 tablespoon oil in workbowl. Process for 60 seconds. Pour ¼ cup oil into pusher that has tiny hole on bottom. Process until oil drips down. Remove pusher, and with machine going, dribble in remaining oil until thickened. Remove cover. Taste. Sprinkle with additional lemon juice and pepper to taste. Process for 5 seconds.

To prepare with electric mayonnaise maker: Combine egg yolk, mustard, lemon juice, salt, and cayenne in machine cup. Proceed, following manufacturer's instructions for adding oil. When whipping is complete, sprinkle with vinegar and stir in pepper to taste, mixing to blend. Mixture will be the consistency of commercial mayonnaise.

All 3 methods prepare mayonnaise that is ready for immediate use. Store remaining mayonnaise in tightly closed jar in refrigerator.

YIELD: About 1 cup

VARIATIONS: Variations are endless; here are a few:

Aromatic Flavor Mayonnaise: Substitute ¼ teaspoon My Spicy Mix (this chapter) for salt.

Tartar Sauce: Stir into finished mayonnaise 2 tablespoons finely minced shallot, ¼ cup well-drained and chopped Bread and Butter Pickles (page 199), 1 tablespoon finely minced parsley, and 2 teaspoons well-rinsed chopped green olives.

Curry Mayonnaise: Add ½ teaspoon mild curry powder and 1 tablespoon minced fresh tarragon, rosemary, or basil (or ½ teaspoon dried variety of any aforementioned herbs) after mixture is completely whipped. Wait 10 minutes before serving.

Aioli (Garlic Mayonnaise): Stir into finished mayonnaise 1 teaspoon finely minced garlic. (Do not use dried garlic.)

Tomato/Chive Mayonnaise: Stir into finished mayonnaise 2 tablespoons finely minced chives and 1 tablespoon tomato puree.

USED IN THESE RECIPES:

Whamburger (10)
Potato Salad (17)
Russian Dressing (19)
Crispy Fish Fillets (34A)
Vegetable Slaw (44)

LIGHT MAYONNAISE

⅔ cup My "Canned" Chicken Broth
    (page 178), or broth made with
    low-sodium vegetable seasoning
1½ teaspoons arrowroot flour
  1 egg yolk
  1 teaspoon prepared Dijon mustard
  1 teaspoon fresh lemon juice
  ¼ teaspoon salt

¼ cup each Italian olive and corn oil
1 teaspoon wine vinegar or apple
  cider vinegar
½ teaspoon dried tarragon or oregano
  leaves, crumbled
1 tablespoon minced fresh parsley or
  dill or a combination of both

1. In cup, combine 2 tablespoons cold broth with arrowroot. Stir to dissolve. Set aside. Heat remaining broth in heavy-bottomed saucepan until simmering. Slowly whisk in arrowroot mixture. Cook briefly until translucent and thickened. Remove from heat. Let cool.
2. *To finish by hand:* In bowl, combine egg yolk, mustard, lemon juice, salt, and 1 tablespoon oil. Whisk until well blended. Slowly dribble in remaining oil a few drops at a time, until half of oil is used. Then pour in a slow, steady stream while whisking, until thickened. Sprinkle with vinegar, tarragon or oregano, and parsley or dill. Whisk again. Whisk in the arrowroot mixture, a little at a time. Mayonnaise will be the consistency of unchilled sour cream.

    To finish in food processor: Fit processor with steel blade. In workbowl, combine egg yolk, mustard, lemon juice, salt, and 1 tablespoon oil. Process for 60 seconds. Pour ¼ cup oil into pusher that has tiny hole in bottom. Process until oil drips down. Pour remaining oil into pusher and process until all oil is incorporated. Uncover, sprinkle with tarragon or oregano and parsley or dill. With machine running, slowly pour arrowroot mixture through feed tube.

    To finish with electric mayonnaise maker: In machine cup, combine egg yolk, mustard, lemon juice, and salt. Proceed, following manufacturer's instructions for adding oil. When whipping is complete, scrape into bowl. Sprinkle with vinegar, tarragon or oregano, and parsley or dill. Whisk to blend. While whisking, slowly add arrowroot mixture.

    Spoon mayonnaise into jar and refrigerate for several hours before using. Mixture will be fairly thick and will thicken further after chilling to spreadable consistency.

YIELD: About 1¼ cups

USED IN THESE RECIPES:

    Whamburger (10)
    Potato Salad (17)
    Crispy Fish Fillets (34A)
    Broccoli-Chicken Salad (71)
    New Coleslaw (90)

Recipes for Healthful "Junk-Food" Clones

The **number in parentheses** corresponds to titles in the list on pages 151–52, from which you can plan your healthful "junk-food" replacements on the Basic All-Family Menu Plan. An **asterisk (*)** means that for a permanent place on that menu plan, the recipe must be converted to an even more healthful one. See the instructions at the end of each recipe. The **letter K** means the recipe is simple enough for your kids to make under your supervision. Recipes are arranged under *Breakfast*, *Lunch*, and *Dinner*.

Healthful "Junk-Food" Clones for Breakfast

*(1)** GRANOLA, THE CEREAL

Serve with ice-cold milk!

2 cups wheat flakes (available in
    health-food stores)
2 cups rolled oats
½ cup unhulled sesame seeds
½ cup shredded unsweetened coconut

½ cup chopped almonds
¾ cup date powder
½ cup regular wheat germ
1 teaspoon ground cinnamon
½ teaspoon salt (optional)

1. In large well-seasoned iron skillet, stir and toast wheat flakes, oats, and sesame seeds, a cup at a time, until seeds start to pop, about 4 minutes. Transfer to large bowl.
2. Add balance of ingredients and stir to combine.

YIELD: About 7¾ cups; recipe may be halved; serving size = ¼ cup

NOTE: For children under 2 years old, pulverize in food blender before serving.

* To CONVERT into an even more healthful recipe eliminate coconut, which is high in saturated fat, and to help compensate for loss of sweetness increase date powder to 1 cup.

(1A)* GRANOLA, THE CEREAL AND SNACK

1 cup unsweetened apple juice
2 tablespoons frozen orange juice
    concentrate
1 teaspoon ground cinnamon
2 tablespoons unsweetened carob
    powder

1 2-inch piece vanilla bean, split
¼ cup peanut or safflower oil
1 recipe Granola (1)

1. In heavy-bottomed saucepan, combine and heat first 5 ingredients to boiling point. Reduce heat to simmering and simmer for 4 to 5 minutes, uncovered, stirring out any clumps of carob. Stir in oil. Let cool. Squeeze out juices from vanilla bean and discard bean. Stir mixture several times.
2. Measure out one-third of granola into bowl. Pour one-third of liquid over granola, tossing to coat. Repeat sequence twice more.
3. Preheat oven to 300°F. Spread granola over 2 jelly-roll pans and bake for 45 minutes, turning with spatula every 10 minutes. Let cool completely.
4. Turn into bowl. Store in tightly sealed glass or tin containers (not plastic). Needs no refrigeration. Mixture will retain its crispiness and flavor for 2 weeks.

YIELD: About 8 cups; serving size = ¼ cup

NOTE: This extra-crisp granola is not recommended for children under 2 years old.

* To convert into an even more healthful recipe, follow the TO CONVERT instructions for the preceding recipe.

(2) CHEWY FRUIT GRANOLA BARS

½ cup each chopped dried unsweetened
    dates, dark raisins, and dried
    apricots (without preservatives
    added)
1 cup unsweetened apple juice
½ teaspoon each ground cinnamon and
    coriander
½ cup rolled oats
¼ cup unhulled sesame seeds
1 cup whole-wheat pastry flour

2 tablespoons unprocessed bran
¼ cup date powder
½ teaspoon salt
½ cup sliced blanched almonds
1 egg
1 tablespoon corn oil
1 tablespoon honey (optional)
1 tablespoon sweet butter/margarine
    blend, melted

1. In heavy-bottomed saucepan, bring dates, raisins, apricots, apple juice, and spices to boil. Reduce heat to simmering. Cover and simmer for 5 minutes. Uncover, and let cool. Pour into large mixing bowl.

2. Spread oats and sesame seeds across heated well-seasoned iron skillet. Toast until seeds start to pop, about 4 minutes, taking care not to burn. Turn into bowl. Stir in flour, bran, date powder, salt, and almonds. Let cool.
3. In cup, beat egg, oil, and optional honey to blend (use honey if you have a particularly sweet tooth). Stir into bowl with cooled fruit mixture. Add oatmeal mix, and beat by hand or with mixing machine for 1 minute, or until combined (do not overbeat).
4. Preheat the oven to 350°F. and grease a 9-inch square baking pan.
5. Spread mixture in pan, smoothing out top with moistened spatula and pushing into corners.
6. Bake for 30 minutes. Brush with melted shortening. Return to oven and bake for 10 minutes. Place on rack and let cool for 30 minutes. With sharp knife, cut into 8 or 10 bars.

YIELD: 8 or 10 bars

(3)K TASTY MUFFINS

2½ cups My Muffin and Cake Mix
  (page 172)
⅓ cup oil
2 eggs
1 tablespoon honey

1 tablespoon frozen orange juice
  concentrate
¾ to 1 cup milk or water or a
  combination of both

1. Place mix in large bowl. In cup, combine oil, eggs, honey, and orange juice concentrate. Blend with fork.
2. Make well in center of mix. Add egg mixture. Then, while stirring, add milk or water a little at a time. Mixture should be thick yet spoonable.
3. Preheat oven to 400° and grease twelve 3-inch muffin cups. Fill cups with batter. Bake for 20 to 25 minutes, or until lightly brown, and toothpick inserted in center comes out clean.

YIELD: 12 muffins

VARIATIONS: Blueberry Muffins: Rinse and pick over 1 cup fresh blueberries. Add ½ teaspoon grated lemon rind. Fold into batter at end of step 2. For extra sweetness without sugar, dissolve 1 tablespoon honey in 1 tablespoon tepid water. Using pastry brush, dab muffins with mixture right after baking.

Banana-Coconut Muffins: Add 3 tablespoons unsweetened shredded coconut to batter at end of step 2. Adjust liquid measurement, if necessary. Fill muffin cups. Coarsely chop ripe banana. Push equal amount of pieces into each batter-filled cup.*

Apricot Muffins: Soak ½ cup dried apricots in water for 30 minutes. Drain, squeezing out liquid. Coarsely chop. Sprinkle equal amounts over muffins and gently press into batter.

Raisin-Bran Muffins: Reduce Muffin and Cake Mix to 2¼ cups. Add ½ cup unprocessed bran and ⅓ cup dark raisins to mix. Increase honey to 2 tablespoons. Use 1¼ to 1½ cups milk instead of water. Dab with honey/water mixture (Blueberry Muffin variation) right after baking.

* To CONVERT into an even more healthful recipe, eliminate coconut, which is high in saturated fat, and substitute 3 tablespoons coarsely chopped walnuts, which contain a healthful fat. Now you have Banana-Nut Muffins.

(4) WONDER-FUL BREAD

3½ to 3¾ *cups unbleached flour*
    1 *package dry yeast*
    1 *teaspoon honey*
    ¾ *cup warm water (105° to*
      115°F.)
    2 *tablespoons nonfat dry milk*
      solids
    ¼ *teaspoon each salt and*
      ground allspice
    ½ *teaspoon ground coriander*
    2 *tablespoons sweet butter/*
      margarine blend, cut into
      pieces

3 *tablespoons plain yogurt*
2 *teaspoons honey*
2 *tablespoons frozen apple*
  juice concentrate
1 *egg white mixed with 1*
  tablespoon water
Unhulled sesame seeds
(optional)

1. In tall glass, combine and blend with fork 2 tablespoons flour, yeast, honey, and ¼ cup warm water. Let stand until mixture rises to top of glass, about 7 minutes.
2. Fit food processor with steel blade. In workbowl, combine 3¼ cups flour, dry milk, salt, spices, and shortening. Process on/off 5 times.
3. Add yeast mixture. Process for 10 seconds. Add yogurt. Process for 10 seconds.
4. Add honey and apple juice concentrate to remaining ½ cup warm water and stir to dissolve, reheating, if necessary. With machine running, slowly pour through feed tube. Process until ball forms and rotates around bowl 15 times. (If dough doesn't congeal and remains sticky, remove cover of processor and sprinkle with remaining flour. Process on/off twice; then process for 15 seconds.) Transfer dough to board and knead briefly. Shape into ball.

5. Lightly oil a large, fairly straight-sided bowl. Drop dough ball in, turning to coat. Cover with plastic wrap. Let rise at room temperature (70° to 80°F.) until double in bulk, about 1¼ hours. Punch down. Knead briefly on board.
6. Cut into 3 equal parts. Shape each piece into ball. Flatten with hands. Using rolling pin, roll each piece into rectangle wide enough to fit loaf pan. Tightly roll up, pinching ends. Lightly grease three mini-loaf pans (5¾" x 3¼" x 2¼") with sweet butter/margarine blend. Group pans together and cover with a single sheet of lightly greased waxed paper.
7. Preheat oven to 375°F. Brush dough with egg wash; sprinkle with sesame seeds, if desired. Bake for 25 to 30 minutes, or until lightly browned. Test for doneness. Remove from pans and tap bottom of loaves with knuckles. A hollow sound indicates loaves are done. If not, place loaves directly on rack in oven and bake for 5 minutes. Let cool completely on rack before slicing.

YIELD: 3 mini-loaves

VARIATION: Change unbleached flour measurement to 3 to 3¼ cups. Add ½ cup stone-ground whole-wheat flour. Finished bread will be more textured.

NOTES: Dough may be cut in half in step 6, shaped into 2 loaves, and baked for 30 to 35 minutes in larger pans (7⅜" x 3⅝" x 2¼").

For soft crust, reduce baking time by 5 minutes, and wrap each fully cooled loaf in plastic wrap. Let stand several hours before slicing.

(5) * BREAKFAST SAUSAGES

¾ *pound boned pork fillets, partially trimmed*
2 *teaspoons My Spicy Mix (page 177)*
¼ *teaspoon freshly grated nutmeg*
½ *teaspoon salt*
⅛ *teaspoon freshly ground black pepper*
1 *tablespoon minced shallot*
2 *teaspoons minced garlic*
3 *whole cloves, crushed*

2 *tablespoons soft bread crumbs or My Shake and Bake-Alike (page 175)*
1 *teaspoon each honey, tomato paste, and apple cider vinegar*
1 *teaspoon oil, plus 1 teaspoon for sautéing*
½ *teaspoon prepared Dijon mustard*
1 *tablespoon finely minced fresh dill*

1. Coarsely grind meat with grinder or food processor. If using food processor, cut meat into 1½-inch cubes. Fit food processor with steel blade. Place meat in workbowl and process on/off until meat is coarsely chopped. (Do not overprocess to paste consistency.) Scrape into bowl.
2. Combine Spicy Mix with nutmeg, salt, and black pepper. Sprinkle over meat. Add shallot, garlic, and cloves and blend.

3. In cup, combine and mash bread crumbs or Shake and Bake-Alike with honey, tomato paste, vinegar, oil, and mustard. Add to meat. Sprinkle with dill. Blend well with hands.
4. Divide mixture into 14 equal parts. Shape into 4-inch sausages by rolling between palms. Arrange in one layer on flat plate. Cover tightly and refrigerate for several hours or overnight to develop flavor.
5. To cook, brush nonstick skillet with 1 teaspoon oil and heat until hot. Over medium heat, lightly brown sausages, uncovered, on all sides for 6 minutes. Reduce heat. Cover and cook for 2 minutes. Drain on paper toweling. Serve very hot.

YIELD: 14 sausages; serving size = 2 sausages

NOTES: Store-bought sausages contain sugar, large amounts of salt, pork fat, and a long list of additives, including indicted carcinogens, nitrates, and nitrites. My delicious sausages are prepared without sugar or additives, and just a minimum of salt and pork fat. A word of caution: beware of chopped or ground pork that's packed in brine and then factory sealed. Use only freshly ground pork—preferably ground in your kitchen (your food processor does a fine job).

Sausages freeze well if tightly wrapped. Partially thaw before cooking; use within 2 weeks.

* To CONVERT into an even more healthful recipe, well trim fillets to remove excess fat.

(6)K PANCAKES

1½ cups My Pancake Mix (page 174)   1 tablespoon frozen orange juice
  1 egg   concentrate
  2 tablespoons oil, plus oil for sautéing   ¼ to ½ cup water
  ¾ cup milk

1. Place mix in bowl. In cup, combine egg, oil, milk, orange juice concentrate, and ¼ cup water. Beat with fork to blend. Add to dry ingredients, and stir until moist. This will make a thick pancake. For a thinner pancake, add remaining ¼ cup water.
2. Prepare pancakes in 3 batches in a nonstick skillet or a well-seasoned iron skillet. Spread ½ teaspoon oil across skillet. Heat until a drop of cold water dropped into skillet bounces off. Pour enough batter into skillet to make four 4-inch pancakes. Cook until bubbles form on top of pancakes. Turn and cook until lightly brown. Transfer to warm plate. Prepare remaining pancakes in the same manner. Leftover batter may be stored in a tightly closed container and refrigerated for up to 2 days. Thin down with water, if necessary, when ready to use.

YIELD: 12 pancakes; serves 4

SERVING SUGGESTIONS: Serve hot from the skillet with honey-sweetened plain yogurt, unsweetened jam, Blueberry Sauce (page 235), or Dessert Topping (page 224).

VARIATIONS: Buckwheat Pancakes: Change Pancake Mix measurement to 1 cup; add ½ cup buckwheat flour.

Blueberry Pancakes: Add 1 cup rinsed and dried blueberries to Basic Pancake or to Buckwheat Pancake variation recipes.

Whole-Wheat Pancakes: Change Pancake Mix measurement to 1 cup; add ½ cup stone-ground whole-wheat flour, 1 teaspoon finely grated orange rind, and ¼ teaspoon ground cinnamon.

Buttermilk Pancakes: Instead of ¾ cup milk, combine 1 cup thick buttermilk (preferably unsalted) with ¼ cup water, adding another ¼ cup water if necessary to make a thick, pourable batter.

Healthful "Junk-Food" Clones for Lunch

(7) CUPPA-SOUP

2 tablespoons Italian olive oil
1½ cups My Frozen Vegetable Mix (page 173)
3 cups My "Canned" Chicken Broth (page 178) or broth made with low-sodium vegetable seasoning
1½ cups canned crushed tomatoes
½ cup potatoes, cut into ¼-inch dice
1 teaspoon balsamic vinegar

⅛ teaspoon each salt and pepper
¼ teaspoon ground marjoram
1 teaspoon dried basil leaves, crushed
½ cup fresh peas
½ cup broken-up thin spaghetti
½ cup well-scrubbed unpeeled zucchini, cut into ½-inch dice
Freshly grated Parmesan cheese

1. Heat oil in 1½- to 2-quart heavy-bottomed saucepan until hot but not smoking. Add Vegetable Mix. Sauté until soft over medium-high heat, about 4 minutes.
2. Add Chicken Broth, tomatoes, potatoes, vinegar, salt, pepper, and herbs. Bring to simmering point. Cover and simmer for 10 minutes.
3. Add peas, spaghetti, and zucchini. Bring to simmering point again. Stir well. Cover and simmer for 20 minutes, stirring from time to time. Remove from heat. Let stand, covered, for 10 minutes. Reheat, if necessary, before serving.
4. Ladle soup into plates, and sprinkle with Parmesan cheese.

YIELD: 5½ to 6 cups; serves 5 to 6

(8)* "CANNED" CUCUMBER-ZUCCHINI SOUP

2 tablespoons Italian olive oil or corn
  oil
1 cup My Frozen Vegetable Mix (page
  173)
1 pound cucumbers, peeled and diced
½ pound zucchini, scrubbed, unpeeled,
  and diced
1 tablespoon apple cider vinegar
2 cups My "Canned" Chicken Broth
  (page 178) or broth made with
  low-sodium vegetable seasoning

1 cup tomato juice
¼ teaspoon each dried dillweed and
  mild curry powder
¼ teaspoon salt
1 tablespoon regular Cream of Wheat
3 tablespoons dairy sour cream or
  plain yogurt

1. Heat oil in 1½- to 2-quart heavy-bottomed saucepan until hot. Add Vegetable Mix, breaking up pieces. Stir and cook over medium-high heat until Vegetable Mix is completely defrosted. Add cucumbers and zucchini. Reduce heat to moderate. Cook until diced vegetables begin to soften, about 4 minutes.
2. Stir in vinegar, cook for 30 seconds. Add Chicken Broth, tomato juice, dill, curry powder, and salt. Bring to simmering point. Sprinkle with Cream of Wheat while stirring. Cover partially and simmer for 25 minutes, stirring once or twice.
3. With bowl underneath, pour into food mill and puree. Discard solids. Whisk in sour cream or yogurt. Reheat to just under boiling point before serving.

YIELD: About 5½ cups; serves 5 to 6

VARIATION: Serve chilled, sprinkled with minced chives and a dollop of sour cream or yogurt on top.

NOTE: If regular tomato juice is used, with salt added, omit ¼ teaspoon salt.

* To CONVERT into an even more healthful recipe, lower fat content by replacing dairy sour cream with low-fat plain yogurt.

(9)K POPCORN

¾ cup popping corn
1 teaspoon oil
3 tablespoons sweet butter/
  margarine blend

1 tablespoon My Seasoning Mix
  (page 176)
1 to 2 tablespoons freshly grated
  Parmesan cheese

1. Pop corn in popcorn maker, or pop as follows: Spread oil onto well-seasoned iron skillet. Heat over medium-high heat for 3 minutes. Sprinkle with corn, spreading out into one layer. Cover and pop, shaking pan around several times until popping ceases. Turn into large bowl.
2. Over low heat, in small heavy-bottomed saucepan, melt butter/margarine blend. Stir in Seasoning Mix. Cook until bubbly. Remove from heat and let stand for 1 minute.
3. While stirring popcorn with large spoon, slowly pour seasoned butter/margarine blend over popcorn until well coated. Sprinkle with cheese to taste and stir again. Serve warm.

YIELD: 1 quart; serving size = ½ cup

SERVING SUGGESTIONS: Use as croutons with soup, and as accompaniments to salads and sandwiches. Take along a batch to the movies!

(10)*K WHAMBURGER

¾ pound lean ground beef
¼ cup My Shake and Bake-Alike (page 175)
¼ cup tomato puree, preferably low-sodium
3 tablespoons finely minced shallot or onion
1 teaspoon finely minced garlic
¼ teaspoon salt

½ teaspoon My Spicy Mix (page 177)
1 tablespoon oil
4 commercial hamburger buns or Hamburger Buns (page 202)
My Real Mayonnaise (page 180)
Thinly sliced cucumber or endive
Thinly sliced tomatoes
Thinly sliced onions

1. In bowl, combine and blend beef with Shake and Bake-Alike, tomato puree, shallots or onion, garlic, and salt. Divide into 4 equal parts. Shape into ¾-inch patties. Sprinkle each patty on both sides with equal amounts of My Spicy Mix, pressing into meat.
   If you're using a skillet: Rub oil across nonstick skillet or well-seasoned iron skillet. Heat until hot but not smoking. Sauté meat, turning every 2 minutes. Cook to desired doneness (7 to 8 minutes for medium rare).
   If you're using a broiler or barbecue: Brush meat lightly with oil. Broil on each side for 4 minutes, or place in barbecue holder and cook over coals, turning every 2 minutes. Cook to desired doneness.
2. Split buns and lightly toast. Spread with mayonnaise. Serve burgers on buns between layers of cucumber or endive, tomatoes, and onions.

YIELD: Serves 4

VARIATION: Whamburgers with Cheese Stuffing: Divide meat into 8 equal parts in step 1. Shape into ⅜-inch patties. In bowl, combine and blend ½ cup shredded sharp cheddar cheese with ½ teaspoon each Worcestershire sauce and prepared Dijon mustard. Spread equal amounts of stuffing over 4 patties. Cover with remaining 4 patties, pinching edges all around to seal. Continue with recipe.

* To CONVERT into an even more healthful recipe, lower fat content by replacing My Real Mayonnaise with Light Mayonnaise (page 182).

(11)* MUSHROOM PIZZA

Dough:

2¼ to 2½ cups unbleached flour, plus
    flour for board
  ½ cup whole-wheat pastry flour
  ¼ teaspoon salt
  2 teaspoons nonfat dry milk
    solids
  1 tablespoon freshly grated
    Parmesan cheese
  1 cup warm water (105° to
    115°F.)
  1 package dry yeast
  2 tablespoons Italian olive oil,
    plus oil for bowl and
    brushing over dough

Sauce:

About 2½ cups warm Pizza
Sauce or Spaghetti Sauce
(page 194)

Topping:

2 tablespoons Italian olive oil
1 medium onion, quartered
  and thinly sliced
2 teaspoons minced garlic
1 sweet green or red pepper,
  seeded, quartered, and
  thinly sliced
½ teaspoon each dried sweet
  basil and oregano leaves
¼ pound snow-white fresh
  mushrooms, ends
  trimmed, rinsed, dried,
  and thinly sliced
3 cups shredded mozzarella
  cheese
½ cups freshly grated
  Parmesan cheese
¼ cup chopped fresh parsley

1. To prepare dough, use food processor fitted with steel blade. Place 2¼ cups unbleached flour, all of whole-wheat flour, salt, dry milk, and Parmesan cheese in workbowl. Process on/off 3 times.
2. Pour warm water into small bowl. Sprinkle with yeast, stirring until dissolved. Add 2 tablespoons oil and stir quickly. With machine running, pour mixture through feed tube and process for 15 seconds. Sprinkle with ¼ cup flour. Process for 10 seconds. Dough will partially clean sides of bowl and will be sticky.
3. Using rubber spatula, scrape onto board sprinkled with 2 tablespoons flour. Knead for about 2 minutes (see Notes), adding another 2 tablespoons flour, if necessary, to make a soft, smooth, elastic dough. (Just the right amount of flour and proper kneading will make a crispy crust.) Shape into ball.

4. Lightly oil fairly straight-sided large bowl. Drop ball into bowl, turning to coat. Cover with plastic wrap. Let rise at room temperature (70° to 80°F.) until puffy and light, 1¾ to 2 hours. Punch down. Cut into 2 pieces. Shape into balls, cover with waxed paper, and refrigerate.
5. Prepare topping by heating oil in well-seasoned iron skillet until hot. Add onion, garlic, sweet pepper, and herbs. Stir and sauté for 2 minutes without browning. Combine mushrooms with mixture, and sauté until all liquid has evaporated.
6. Preheat oven to 450°F. and lightly grease two 10-inch pie pans or pizza pans. Lightly flour board. Roll each ball of dough into a ¼-inch-thick circle. Put dough into pans and brush with oil. Bake for 5 minutes. Remove from oven, leaving oven on.
7. To assemble, spread each just-prepared pizza shell with ¾ cup warm sauce. Top with mozzarella cheese; dribble with remaining sauce. Then sprinkle with Parmesan cheese, parsley, and topping. Bake on lowest rack in already-hot oven for 15 to 20 minutes, or until cheese is bubbly and shell is crisp. Cut into wedges with pizza cutter or sharp shears, and serve immediately.

YIELD: 2 pizzas; 4 to 6 wedges per pizza

VARIATIONS: Variations are endless. Here are a few: Add to topping in step 5 sautéed tiny meatballs, sautéed chicken pieces, rare cooked beef or pork pieces, cubed tofu, lightly sautéed shrimp, broken up and lightly sautéed Breakfast Sausages (page 187).

NOTES: If low-sodium tomato products are used, add ¼ teaspoon salt in step 5, if desired.

Here's how to knead: Push the dough down and then forward with heel of your hand; then fold the dough over toward you. Make a quarter turn, and push and fold as before. Repeat turning, pushing, and folding until the texture of the dough becomes smooth and elastic, and can be easily shaped into a nonsticky ball.

* To CONVERT into an even more healthful recipe, lower fat content by reducing mozzarella cheese to 1½ cups. Keep flavor high by increasing dried basil and oregano to ¾ teaspoon each, and adding a pinch of salt to topping if desired. Also use converted versions of Pizza Sauce or Spaghetti Sauce (look for the asterisk at the end of the recipes).

(12)*K PIZZA SAUCE

2 tablespoons Italian olive oil
1 cup My Frozen Vegetable Mix (page 173)
¼ pound snow-white fresh mushrooms, ends trimmed, rinsed, dried, and coarsely chopped
1 2-pound 3-ounce can Italian tomatoes with basil

¼ teaspoon salt
1 bay leaf, wrapped in washed cotton cheesecloth and tied with white cotton thread
3 tablespoons tomato paste, preferably without added salt
2 teaspoons dried oregano leaves, crushed

1. In 2-quart heavy-bottomed saucepan, heat oil over moderately high heat until hot but not smoking. Add Vegetable Mix. Cook and stir until most of liquid evaporates. Add mushrooms. Cook for 3 minutes, stirring often.
2. Stir in tomatoes, breaking up with large spoon. Add remaining ingredients and combine. Bring to boil. Reduce heat to simmering, and simmer, uncovered, for 30 minutes, stirring from time to time. Remove from heat. Stir. Cover and let stand for 10 minutes. Discard bay leaf bundle.

YIELD: About 4½ cups; serving size = ¾ cup

VARIATION: Add 1 teaspoon tarragon vinegar and ½ teaspoon curry powder in step 2. Wonderful new flavor!

NOTE: If tomatoes prepared with basil are not available, substitute ⅓ cup tightly packed minced fresh basil, or 1½ teaspoons dried basil leaves, crushed, to unseasoned canned tomatoes. Fresh basil, though, is preferable.

* To CONVERT into an even more healthful recipe, reduce salt content by using canned Italian tomatoes with basil, no salt added, and adding ⅛ teaspoon salt.

(13)* SPAGHETTI SAUCE

1 small carrot, peeled and trimmed
2 medium onions
1 small sweet green or red pepper, seeded
2 large cloves garlic
3 tablespoons Italian olive oil
1 pound lean ground beef
1½ teaspoons each dried oregano and basil leaves, crushed
¼ teaspoon salt

⅛ teaspoon cayenne pepper (optional)
2 teaspoons wine vinegar or balsamic vinegar
1 2-pound can Italian tomatoes
1 6-ounce can tomato paste, preferably without salt added
1½ cups My "Canned" Chicken Broth (page 178) or broth made with low-sodium vegetable seasoning

1. Use food processor to chop vegetables. Cut carrot, onions, and green or red pepper into uniform pieces. Halve garlic cloves. Fit food processor with steel blade. Place cut ingredients in workbowl. Process on/off about 4 times, or until mixture is finely chopped (take care not to puree).
2. Heat oil in well-seasoned iron skillet until hot. Sauté vegetable mixture until wilted but not brown, stirring constantly.
3. Add meat, breaking up pieces with large spoon. Sprinkle with herbs and spices. Stir and sauté until lightly browned and all liquid has evaporated. Pour vinegar around sides of skillet. Cook for 1 minute.
4. Partially puree tomato solids (reserving liquid) and tomato paste in food processor. Pour into skillet. Add reserved liquid from can and Chicken Broth. Bring to boil. Reduce heat to simmering. Partially cover and simmer for 1¼ hours, stirring from time to time.

YIELD: About 6¼ cups; serving size = ¾ cup

VARIATION: If you have Breakfast Sausages (page 187) on hand, use 4 of them, and reduce ground meat weight to ¾ pound.

* To CONVERT into an even more healthful recipe, reduce the salt content by using canned Italian tomatoes, no salt added, and adding ⅛ teaspoon salt.

(14) FISH AND SHRIMP STICKS

1 egg
1 tablespoon each fresh lemon juice
    and water
1 teaspoon corn or peanut oil
¼ teaspoon each salt and onion powder
3 tablespoons cornstarch
½ cup fine bread crumbs, preferably
    homemade (page 217), or My
    Shake and Bake-Alike (page 175)

½ pound medium shrimp, shelled,
    deveined, and well dried
½ pound thick scrod fillet, cut into ½-
    inch strips
4 tablespoons peanut oil
Minced fresh parsley
½ lemon, plus lemon wedges for
    garnish

1. Place egg, lemon juice, water, 1 teaspoon peanut oil, salt, and onion powder in shallow dish and beat with fork to blend. Set aside.
2. Tear off 2 large sheets of waxed paper. On one sheet, spread out cornstarch; on another sheet, spread out bread crumbs or Shake and Bake-Alike.
3. Coat shrimp and fish sticks individually in cornstarch, shaking off excess. Then dip them in egg mixture, coating well. Dredge each piece in crumbs or Shake and Bake-Alike, pressing to hold crumbs. Chill in freezer for 10 minutes.
4. Use 2 nonstick skillets so that shrimp and fish sticks may be cooked in one layer without crowding. Heat 1 tablespoon oil in nonstick skillet. Start to

cook fish sticks first, as they require more cooking time, arranging fish in one layer. Cook on one side until lightly browned, about 4 minutes. Add another tablespoon oil and turn.
5. Start cooking shrimp in second skillet after turning fish sticks. Heat 1 table-spoon oil in nonstick skillet, arranging shrimp in one layer. Cook until lightly browned, 2½ to 3 minutes. Turn. Add remaining tablespoon oil. Cook until delicately browned (do not overcook or shrimp will become tough).
6. Arrange fish sticks and shrimp on platter. Sprinkle with parsley and lemon juice, and garnish with lemon wedges.

YIELD: Serves 4

(15)* CREAMED MUSHROOMS

1 teaspoon Italian olive oil
4 teaspoons sweet butter/
   margarine blend
2 tablespoons minced shallot
¼ pound snow-white fresh
   mushrooms, ends trimmed,
   rinsed, dried, and coarsely
   chopped
5 teaspoons unbleached flour
1½ teaspoons My Spicy Mix
   (page 177)
About ¾ cup My "Canned" Chicken
   Broth (page 178) or broth
   made with low-sodium
   vegetable seasoning

3 tablespoons cream
2 to 3 tablespoons tomato puree
2 tablespoons finely grated
   sharp cheddar cheese or
   freshly grated Parmesan
   cheese
2 tablespoons minced fresh
   parsley or dill
Pinch salt

1. Heat oil and butter/margarine blend in heavy-bottomed saucepan (prefer-ably enameled). Add shallot and mushrooms. Sauté over medium heat until wilted, about 5 minutes, stirring constantly, and taking care not to brown.
2. Sprinkle with flour and My Spicy Mix, stirring constantly. Mixture will become very thick. Stir and cook for 1 minute without browning, adding chicken broth a little at a time. Bring to simmering point.
3. In cup combine cream with 2 tablespoons tomato puree and add to sauce. Stir. Add cheese and parsley or dill. Cook, uncovered, for 5 minutes over very low heat, stirring often.
4. Taste. If desired, add remaining tomato puree and pinch of salt.

YIELD: About 1⅓ cups; serving size = ⅓ cup

SERVING SUGGESTIONS: Serve over steamed vegetables, fish, cooked chicken or meat, or just-made toast.

NOTE: Additional chicken broth may be added at the end of step 3 if a thinner sauce is desired.

* To CONVERT into an even more healthful recipe, reduce fat content by replacing cream with whole milk; reduce Parmesan cheese to 1 tablespoon and use instead of Cheddar.

(16)K   FRENCH FRIES

3 medium baking potatoes (about 1 pound), peeled, cut into ⅜-inch strips
2 tablespoons Italian olive or corn oil
3 tablespoons minced shallots

1½ teaspoons minced garlic (optional)
1 teaspoon My Spicy Mix (page 177)
1¼ teaspoons balsamic or red wine vinegar

1. Preheat oven to 450°F. Lay cut potatoes on paper toweling. Dry well.
2. Brush oil over jelly-roll pan. Place pan in oven for 5 minutes. Add potatoes in one layer. Sprinkle with shallots, garlic, and Spicy Mix, turning with spatula several times to evenly coat. Bake for 5 minutes, and turn. Bake for another 5 minutes.
3. Sprinkle with vinegar, turning several times with spatula. Turn oven heat up to 475°F. Bake potatoes for 8 to 10 minutes more, or until lightly browned and tender. Serve immediately.

YIELD: Serves 4

VARIATION: In step 3, omit vinegar; sprinkle potatoes with 1 tablespoon freshly grated Parmesan cheese.

(17) *   POTATO SALAD

1½ *pounds red-skinned potatoes (see*
    Note)
1 *small carrot*
1 *medium onion*
1 *small sweet red pepper, seeded*
2 *small ribs celery, trimmed*
1 *large clove garlic*
3 *tablespoons wine vinegar*
2 *tablespoons Italian olive oil*
3 *tablespoons My "Canned"*
    Chicken Broth (page 178) or
    broth made with low-sodium
    vegetable seasoning

1 *teaspoon prepared Dijon mustard*
1 *tablespoon My Spicy Mix (page*
    177)
3 to 4 *tablespoons My Real Mayonnaise*
    (page 180)
2 *tablespoons minced fresh parsley*
    Freshly ground black pepper

1. In heavy-bottomed saucepan, cook potatoes in rapidly boiling water to cover until tender, about 20 minutes. Drain. Let stand until cool enough to handle. Peel and quarter each potato. Place in large bowl.
2. Cut carrot, onion, red pepper, celery, and garlic into uniform pieces. Place in workbowl of food processor that has been fitted with steel blade, and process on/off 3 to 4 times until coarsely chopped. Measure out 1 cup of mixture and set aside. Reserve any remaining mixture for soup or salads.
3. In cup, combine vinegar, olive oil, Chicken Broth, and mustard. Beat with fork to blend. Pour over slightly warm potatoes. Gently toss briefly. Sprinkle with Spicy Mix; stir in mayonnaise.
4. Chill for several hours before serving, stirring once or twice. Sprinkle with parsley and freshly ground pepper.

YIELD: About 3 cups; serves 6

NOTE: Red-skinned potatoes have been selected for their natural sweetness and delicate flavor, but any other firm potato may be used with delicious results. Peel and cut them into 1-inch cubes before cooking.

* To CONVERT into an even more healthful recipe, reduce fat content by substituting Light Mayonnaise (page 182) for My Real Mayonnaise, adding after chilling (step 4).

(18)*K   BREAD AND BUTTER PICKLES

2 pounds Kirby cucumbers, well
     scrubbed, ends trimmed, thinly
     sliced
2 tablespoons finely minced shallot
1 teaspoon finely minced garlic
4 large sprigs dill, including thick
     stems
3 tablespoons pickling spices

2 cups apple cider vinegar
1½ teaspoons salt
½ teaspoon each ground ginger and
     freshly grated nutmeg
1 tablespoon sugar
2 tablespoons honey
     Pinch crushed red pepper

1. Place cucumbers, shallot, garlic, and dill sprigs in large bowl.
2. Make loose spice bundle by enclosing pickling spices in piece of washed cotton cheesecloth secured with white thread.
3. In heavy-bottomed saucepan, combine vinegar and balance of ingredients. Drop in spice bundle. Bring to boil. Reduce heat to simmering. Partially cover and simmer for 10 minutes. Pour over cucumbers (include the bundle). Let cool, uncovered, stirring and spooning cucumbers with liquid several times. Squeeze out liquid from bundle.
4. Drop bundle into 1-quart jar. Transfer pickles, dill sprigs, and juices to jar. Cover tightly. Refrigerate for at least 2 days before serving, inverting jar from time to time while flavors develop. Pickles will keep in refrigerator for up to 2 weeks.

YIELD: 1 quart; serving size = up to ½ cup

NOTE: If you prefer to store pickles in two 1-pint jars, prepare 2 loose spice bundles in step 2 and drop one bundle in each jar in step 4.

* To CONVERT into an even more healthful recipe eliminate sugar; to maintain sweetness reduce vinegar to 1¾ cups and increase honey to 3 tablespoons.

(19)K   KETCHUP DE-LITE

1 cup tomato puree
2 tablespoons tomato paste
1 tablespoon Italian olive or corn oil
½ teaspoon ground ginger
1½ teaspoons apple cider vinegar

2 teaspoons honey
1 tablespoon minced fresh parsley
⅛ teaspoon cayenne pepper
¼ teaspoon salt (optional)

1. Place tomato puree and tomato paste in bowl. Beat with whisk to blend. Add balance of ingredients, one at a time, whisking after each addition. Cover and let stand for 30 minutes before using.
2. Refrigerate in tightly closed jar. Ketchup will keep in refrigerator for up to 2 weeks.

YIELD: About 1¼ cups; serving size = up to 4 tablespoons

VARIATIONS: Add ½ teaspoon chili powder or chili con carne seasoning and 2 tablespoons chopped shallot or onion.

Russian Dressing: Combine equal amounts of Ketchup De-Lite with My Real Mayonnaise (page 180).

(20) BARBECUE KETCHUP

¼ cup My ''Canned'' Chicken Broth (page 178) or broth made with low-sodium vegetable seasoning
2 medium onions, cut up
4 large sprigs parsley, florets only
⅛ teaspoon each salt and freshly ground black pepper
¼ teaspoon ground ginger and freshly grated nutmeg

⅛ teaspoon cayenne pepper
½ teaspoon chili con carne seasoning
2 tablespoons honey
1 tablespoon Italian olive or corn oil
1 cup tomato puree
2 tablespoons tomato paste, preferably no salt added
½ teaspoon Worcestershire sauce
1½ teaspoons fresh lemon juice

1. Fit food processor with steel blade. In workbowl, combine broth, onions, and parsley. Process until pureed. Scrape into small, heavy-bottomed saucepan. Add salt and spices. Simmer, uncovered, until most of liquid evaporates, stirring from time to time.
2. Remove from heat and stir in balance of ingredients. Pour into glass jar. Cover tightly and chill for at least 1 hour before serving. Ketchup will retain its freshness in refrigerator for up to 7 days.

YIELD: About 1½ cups; serving size = up to 3 tablespoons

NOTE: Proportion of seasonings may be adjusted to your taste buds.

*(21)**   MY REAL MAYONNAISE
(See page 180)

* For an even more healthful mayonnaise, see Light Mayonnaise, page 182.

(22)K   SALAD DRESSING

⅓ cup balsamic vinegar or red wine
  vinegar
⅓ cup tomato juice, preferably low-
  sodium (see Note)
⅓ cup Italian olive oil
1½ teaspoons My Spicy Mix (page
  177) or My Seasoning Mix
  (page 176)

2 tablespoons fresh lemon juice
1 tablespoon finely minced shallot
¼ teaspoon salt (optional)

1. Combine all ingredients in jar and shake well.
2. Let stand at room temperature for 30 minutes before serving. Store in refrigerator.

YIELD: A little more than 1 cup; serving size = 2 tablespoons

NOTE: I choose the low-sodium variety of tomato juice because of its pure
natural tomato flavor. If you prefer the regular variety with added salt, omit
the ¼ teaspoon salt.

(23)*K   CHEESE BUTTER

1 teaspoon prepared Dijon mustard,
  preferably without salt
1 tablespoon tomato puree or Ketchup
  De-Lite (page 199)
⅛ teaspoon freshly grated nutmeg
1 tablespoon fresh lemon juice
¼ pound sweet butter/margarine blend,
  partially softened

3 tablespoons finely minced fresh
  parsley
⅓ cup finely grated sharp cheddar
  cheese
⅛ teaspoon each salt and cayenne
  pepper
2 teaspoons finely minced shallot or
  onion

1. In small bowl, combine and whisk mustard, tomato puree or Ketchup De-
   Lite, nutmeg, and lemon juice.
2. Place butter/margarine blend, parsley, and cheese in shallow dish and mash
   with fork. Blend in mustard mixture, then stir in salt, cayenne pepper, and
   shallot or onion.
3. Pile into jar. Cover tightly and refrigerate. Let flavors ripen for 1 hour before
   using.

YIELD: ¾ cup (recipe may be doubled); serving size = up to 1 tablespoon

SERVING SUGGESTIONS: Serve over hot vegetables, as a spread, or use in place
of butter when preparing fish.

* To CONVERT into an even more healthful recipe, reduce fat content by substituting 3 tablespoons freshly grated Parmesan cheese for ⅓ cup cheddar.

(24) HAMBURGER BUNS

3 cups unbleached flour
3 teaspoons plus 1 tablespoon
   honey
1 package dry yeast
¾ to 1 cup warm water (105° to
   115°F.)
½ cup stone-ground whole-wheat
   flour

½ teaspoon salt
¼ teaspoon ground cinnamon
1 tablespoon nonfat dry milk
   solids
⅓ cup corn or peanut oil
2 eggs
Unhulled sesame seeds
   (optional)

1. In tall glass, combine and blend with fork, 2 tablespoons unbleached flour, 1 teaspoon honey, yeast, and ¼ cup warm water. Let stand until mixture rises to top of glass, about 7 minutes.
2. Fit food processor with steel blade. In workbowl, combine 2¾ cups unbleached flour, all of whole-wheat flour, salt, cinnamon, dry milk, and 2 teaspoons honey. Sprinkle with oil. Process on/off 4 times.
3. Add yeast mixture. Process until blended, about 10 seconds.
4. In cup, combine 1 tablespoon honey and 1 egg. With machine running, pour mixture through feed tube. Process for 3 seconds. Then start processor again and dribble in enough remaining warm water to make a soft, smooth nonsticky ball. Process until ball rotates around workbowl 10 to 12 times. If dough is still sticky, sprinkle board with remaining 2 tablespoons unbleached flour. Transfer dough to board, and knead briefly until dough is no longer sticky. Shape into ball.
5. Lightly oil a large, fairly straight-sided bowl, and drop dough in. Turn to coat. Cover with plastic wrap and let rise at room temperature (70° to 80°F.) until double in bulk, about 1 hour. Punch down. Knead briefly, squeezing out bubbles. Cut in half; then cut each half into 6 equal pieces. Cover with plastic wrap and let rest for 5 minutes.
6. Lightly grease 2 baking sheets and 2 sheets waxed paper. Shape each dough piece into smooth ball and place on sheets. With palm of hand flatten balls to 3½-inch diameter. Cover with waxed paper and let stand until doubled, about 50 minutes.
7. Preheat oven to 375°F. In cup, beat remaining egg with 1 tablespoon water. Using pastry brush, brush each bun with egg wash. Sprinkle with sesame seeds, if desired. Bake for 12 to 15 minutes, or until lightly browned. (If you like your buns crunchy, bake for 20 minutes.) Cool on rack.

YIELD: 12 buns

SERVING SUGGESTION: Split and use as a sandwich bread. Toast, if desired.

VARIATION: Dough makes excellent loaves, too. For 2 loaves, cut dough in half at end of step 5. Shape each half into ball. Flatten with hands. Using rolling pin, roll each piece into rectangle wide enough to fit loaf pan. Tightly roll up, pinching ends. Place seam down in 2 lightly greased 7⅜" x 3⅝" x 2¼" pans. Cover with greased sheet of waxed paper and let rise until well above sides of pan. Brush with egg wash, and sprinkle with sesame seeds, if desired. Bake for about 35 minutes in preheated 375°F. oven. Test for doneness: Remove from pans and tap bottom of loaves with knuckles. A hollow sound indicates loaves are done. Let loaves cool completely before slicing.

(25)K APPLESAUCE

2 pounds crisp sweet apples, scrubbed,
    cored, and sliced
2 tablespoons frozen orange juice
    concentrate

1 cup unsweetened apple juice
½ teaspoon ground cinnamon
3 dashes ground allspice
    Honey to taste (optional)

1. Combine first 3 ingredients in heavy-bottomed 2½- to 3-quart saucepan. Bring to boil. Reduce heat to simmering. Cover and cook until apples are tender, about 12 minutes (cooking time may vary with texture and ripeness of apples). Remove from heat. Let stand, uncovered, for 15 minutes.
2. Puree in food mill. While warm, stir in cinnamon, allspice, and honey, if desired.

YIELD: 2½ cups; serving size = ½ cup

VARIATION: Add ¼ teaspoon ground cardamom in beginning of step 1.

(26)* BROWN SUGAR COOKIES

2¼ cups My Muffin and Cake Mix
    (page 172)
¼ teaspoon baking soda
¼ teaspoon each ground ginger and
    cinnamon
¼ cup each finely chopped walnuts
    and coarsely chopped walnuts
¼ pound sweet butter/margarine
    blend, cut into pieces

¾ cup date powder
2 tablespoons dark brown sugar
1 teaspoon pure vanilla extract
2 teaspoons unsulphured blackstrap
    molasses
1 egg

1. In bowl, combine Muffin and Cake Mix with baking soda, spices, and the finely chopped walnuts. Stir to combine. Set aside.
2. Using mixing machine, combine in mixing bowl, shortening, date powder, dark brown sugar, vanilla, and molasses. Beat on medium speed until creamy and light, stopping machine twice to scrape down sides of bowl. Add egg and beat until blended.

3. With machine going on slow speed, add dry ingredients, ½ cup at a time. Increase speed to medium, and add coarsely chopped walnuts. Beat until mixture is soft and crumbly.
4. With hands, gather mixture up in 4 parts, squeezing each part with palms into 4 balls. Shape each ball into a 4-inch-long log. Place each log on a sheet of waxed paper and roll up tightly, twisting ends of paper to secure. Freeze overnight.
5. Remove from freezer and let stand at room temperature for 20 minutes (do not defrost entirely). Cut with sharp knife into ⅛-inch slices. Arrange on ungreased cookie sheet, 16 cookies at a time, and bake at 375°F. for 12 minutes, or until lightly browned. Transfer to plate and let cookies cool completely before serving. Store in tightly closed tin.

YIELD: 64 cookies

NOTE: Frozen dough may be stored in freezer for 2 weeks; baked cookies will stay crisp in tin for up to 10 days.

* To CONVERT into an even more healthful recipe while maintaining sweetness, use converted Muffin and Cake Mix, eliminate brown sugar, and increase date powder to ¾ cup plus 2 tablespoons.

(27)*K OATMEAL COOKIES

¾ cup unbleached flour	½ cup date powder
½ teaspoon baking soda	3 tablespoons firmly packed brown sugar
¼ teaspoon salt	
2 tablespoons regular wheat germ	1 teaspoon pure vanilla extract
2⅓ cups regular rolled oats pulverized with food processor or blender	1 egg
	3 tablespoons frozen apple juice concentrate
½ teaspoon ground cinnamon	
¼ teaspoon freshly grated nutmeg	⅓ cup coarsely chopped walnuts
¼ cup sweet butter/margarine blend	

1. In bowl, combine and blend first 7 ingredients. Set aside.
2. In large bowl of mixing machine, combine shortening, date powder, brown sugar, and vanilla. Beat on medium speed until well blended.
3. In cup, place egg and apple juice concentrate. Beat with fork. Add to batter and beat for 1 minute.
4. While beating, add dry ingredients, a ¼ cup at a time. Then briefly beat in nuts. Mixture will be very thick.
5. Preheat oven to 350°F. Drop by spoonfuls onto cookie sheets, arranging 16 per sheet. With moistened fork press each cookie to ¼-inch thickness. Bake for 12 to 15 minutes, taking care that cookies don't burn. Cool on rack.

6. Cookies can be served slightly warm (they'll be deliciously sweet-tasting), or at room temperature. Cool completely before storing in a tightly covered tin. They're excellent keepers.

YIELD: About 4 dozen cookies

* To CONVERT into an even more healthful recipe, omit sugar, maintaining sweetness by increasing date powder to ⅔ cup.

*(28) *K CRUNCHY CANDY BALLS*

1 8-ounce package cream cheese
4 tablespoons unsalted peanut butter
½ teaspoon each ground coriander and cinnamon
¼ teaspoon ground ginger
2 teaspoons nonfat dry milk solids

1 teaspoon frozen orange or apple juice concentrate
½ cup Granola (1) page 183, or see variation below
1 teaspoon honey (optional)

1. In small bowl, combine cream cheese with peanut butter, spices, and milk solids. Mash with fork to blend.
2. Blend in juice concentrate; then add Granola. Mix until thoroughly blended. Taste. Add honey if more sweetness is desired. Blend again.
3. Shape into balls the diameter of a quarter. Arrange on flat plate in one layer. Cover with waxed paper and chill.

YIELD: 16 balls

VARIATION: If Granola is not already on your shelf, substitute ¼ cup each date powder and pan-toasted unsweetened Familia (a Swiss dry cereal available in supermarkets). For children under 2 years old, pulverize in blender before using.

* To CONVERT into an even more healthful recipe, reduce fat content by substituting 8 ounces well-drained dry-curd cottage cheese for cream cheese. Also use converted Granola recipe, adding a sprinkling of salt, if desired. The texture will be different, but you'll like it.

*(29) *K 3-JUICE JELL-O OR POPSICLES*

1 6-ounce can unsweetened pineapple juice
¾ cup unsweetened dark grape juice

½ cup unsweetened apple juice
1 tablespoon sugar
1 package unflavored gelatin

1. In saucepan, bring the 3 juices to boil. Stir in sugar.
2. Place gelatin in medium bowl. Add hot fruit juices and stir until gelatin is completely dissolved.

3. Pour into dessert dishes or Popsicle molds. Chill dessert dishes until set; freeze Popsicles.

YIELD: Jell-O serves 4; 6 to 8 Popsicles

VARIATION: Chill mixture until it is the consistency of unbeaten egg whites. Stir in ½ cup pureed fresh fruit, or 1 cup chopped fresh fruit or whole berries. Chill until firm. Serves 6.

* To CONVERT into an even more healthful recipe, eliminate sugar and replace with 2 tablespoons honey.

(30)* PEACH ICE CREAM

1½ cups milk
½ cup cream
½ teaspoon ground coriander
1 1-inch piece vanilla bean, split
1 egg
2 tablespoons sugar

1 teaspoon cornstarch dissolved in 1 teaspoon water
2 tablespoons honey
3 ripe peaches, peeled and coarsely chopped

1. Bring water in bottom of double boiler to boil. Reduce heat to simmering. In top of double boiler combine and stir milk, cream, coriander, and vanilla bean. Cook until just below boiling point. Remove from heat.
2. In cup, combine and blend egg and sugar with fork. Pour in a thin stream into hot milk mixture while stirring. Place over simmering water. Cook for 5 minutes, whisking from time to time.
3. Dribble in cornstarch mixture while whisking. Cook until mixture coats metal spoon. Remove from heat. Press out juices from vanilla bean, and discard bean. Let cool, whisking occasionally. Stir in honey and peaches.
4. Pour into ice-cream maker, following manufacturer's directions, or pour into empty ice-cube trays. Turn refrigerator up to its coldest setting. Cover tray, and freeze, stirring from time to time. After 1 hour, vigorously stir with wooden spoon. Return tray to freezer until mixture sets to desired consistency.

YIELD: About 1 pint; serving size = ½ cup

* To CONVERT into an even more healthful recipe while maintaining flavor, reduce fat content by eliminating cream and increasing milk to 2 cups; and eliminating sugar, increasing honey to 3 tablespoons, and adding ⅛ teaspoon ground cinnamon.

(31)* BLACK CHERRY–BANANA ICE CREAM

1½ cups milk
 ½ cup cream
 1 2-inch piece vanilla bean, split
 2 tablespoons black cherry concentrate
   (available in health-food stores)
 2 tablespoons My Fruit Butter (page
   178)

Dash salt
2 egg yolks
1 ripe medium banana, mashed
1 tablespoon honey

1. Bring water in bottom of double boiler to boil. Reduce heat to simmering. In top of double boiler, combine and stir first 6 ingredients. Cook until just below boiling point.
2. In cup, lightly beat egg yolks with fork. Pour about ¼ cup hot liquid into cup and blend. Pour mixture back into pot and cook until it coats back of spoon, about 4 minutes. Stir in banana. Press out juices from vanilla bean and discard bean. Let cool, stirring occasionally. Stir in honey.
3. Pour into ice-cream maker, following manufacturer's directions, or pour into empty ice-cube trays. Turn refrigerator up to its coldest setting. Cover tray, and freeze, stirring from time to time. After 1 hour, briskly whisk or beat with portable electric beater or rotary mixer. Return tray to freezer until ice cream sets to desired consistency.

YIELD: About 1 pint; serving size = ½ cup

* To CONVERT into an even more healthful recipe while maintaining flavor, eliminate cream and increase milk to 2 cups.

(32) CHEWY BROWNIES

3 tablespoons unsweetened
   carob powder
8 ounces dried unsweetened
   dates, chopped
1 teaspoon baking soda
½ cup each water and
   unsweetened apple juice
2¼ to 2½ cups unbleached flour
1 teaspoon ground cinnamon
¼ teaspoon freshly grated
   nutmeg

3 tablespoons sweet butter/
   margarine blend
⅓ cup date powder
2 tablespoons honey
2 eggs
½ cup plain yogurt
⅓ cup coarsely chopped
   walnuts
½ teaspoon pure vanilla extract
1 teaspoon sweet butter/
   margarine blend, melted

1. In bowl, combine carob, dates, and baking soda.
2. Bring water and apple juice to boil. Pour over dates, stirring well (mixture will foam up). Let stand until cooled.
3. Into bowl, sift flour, cinnamon, and nutmeg. Set aside.

4. In large bowl of mixing machine, place shortening, date powder, and honey. Beat on medium speed until blended. Add eggs. Beat for 1 minute; scrape down sides of bowl. Add yogurt and beat for 30 seconds. While beating, add cooled date mixture, a little at a time, until blended.
5. Beat in dry ingredients, ½ cup at a time, using enough to produce a thick, spoonable batter. Add nuts and vanilla, and beat for 30 seconds.
6. Preheat the oven to 375°F. and grease a 9-inch square baking pan. Evenly spread the batter in the pan and bake for 45 to 50 minutes. When cake starts to come away from sides of pan and toothpick inserted into center comes out slightly moist, remove from oven. Brush with shortening.
7. Let pan cool on rack for 15 minutes. Cut into 16 squares. Serve slightly warm or at room temperature. Freeze leftovers.

YIELD: 16 brownies

NOTE: A frozen Chewy Brownie, placed in your child's lunchbox in the morning, will be defrosted and ready to enjoy by lunchtime.

Healthful "Junk-Food" Clones for Dinner

(33)* "CANNED" TOMATO SOUP

2 tablespoons oil
2 tablespoons minced shallot
2 cups My "Canned" Chicken Broth (page 178) or broth made with low-sodium vegetable seasoning
2 cups canned tomatoes
2 tablespoons unsweetened apple juice
¼ teaspoon each freshly grated nutmeg, dried tarragon leaves, crushed, and salt

1 bay leaf
½ cup cream or equal amounts of cream and milk
2 tablespoons arrowroot flour dissolved in 2 tablespoons water (see Note)
½ cup cooked brown rice
2 teaspoons honey (optional)
Freshly ground black pepper to taste
1 tablespoon minced fresh parsley or dill

1. In 1½- to 2-quart heavy-bottomed saucepan, heat oil until hot. Add shallot and sauté over medium heat until wilted but not brown, stirring continually.
2. Add broth, tomatoes, apple juice, nutmeg, tarragon, salt, and bay leaf. Bring to boil. Reduce heat to simmering. Cover and simmer for 15 minutes.

3. Pour soup into food mill with bowl underneath and puree. Return puree to saucepan over low heat. Whisk in cream. Bring to simmering point. While whisking, dribble in half of arrowroot mixture, and cook until soup begins to thicken. Add remaining arrowroot if you prefer a thicker consistency.
4. Stir in rice. Heat until just under simmering point. Taste. Add honey if you prefer a slightly sweet flavor, and pepper to taste. Serve hot or chilled, sprinkled with parsley or dill.

YIELD: 4 cups; serves 4

NOTE: Soup thickens as it cools. If you're planning to serve cold, use half of arrowroot mixture.

* To CONVERT into an even more healthful recipe, reduce fat content by replacing cream with milk.

(34) THREE TV DINNERS

FISH DINNER
CHICKEN DINNER
MEXICAN DINNER

These TV dinners look like the frozen TV dinners you buy in the supermarket, but that's where the resemblance ends. These are healthful and nutritious. Here's how to make them look like their commercial counterparts by creating your own TV-dinner pans:

Use four 3-compartment disposable ovenproof pans, or fashion your own pans by using four 8-inch pans into which 2 individual large cupcake pans or dishes are inserted. The main dish goes into the larger compartment; the accompanying dishes (vegetables, potatoes, rice, and so forth) into the smaller ones.

All dishes freeze beautifully with the exception of the salsa in the Mexican Dinner, which is not freezeable; so have fun preparing it the same day, or the day before, you go Mexican.

(34A) *Fish Dinner*

(Crispy Fish Fillets, Creamy Mashed Potatoes, Colorful Mixed Vegetables)

* CRISPY FISH FILLETS

1¼ *pounds thin flounder fillets, each*
  fillet cut in half (see Note)
2 *tablespoons fresh lemon juice*
2 *teaspoons frozen orange juice*
  concentrate
¼ *cup evaporated milk*
⅛ *teaspoon salt*

1 *cup My Shake and Bake-Alike (page*
  175)
2 *tablespoons peanut or corn oil*
  Lemon wedges
  My Real Mayonnaise (page 180)
  (optional)

1. Wash fish thoroughly and dry with paper toweling. Place in rectangular baking dish. Spread out into one layer. Sprinkle with lemon juice turning to coat. Marinate for 15 minutes.
2. In shallow bowl, combine orange juice concentrate, milk, and salt. Beat with fork to blend.
3. Sprinkle half of Shake and Bake-Alike across sheet of waxed paper. Dip each fillet into orange juice mixture, then lay atop Shake and Bake-Alike, pressing to adhere. Sprinkle fish with remaining ½ cup of mix and press to adhere. Cover with another sheet of waxed paper. Lay package on plate and place in freezer for 10 to 15 minutes to set.
4. Using large nonstick skillet, heat 1 tablespoon oil until hot. Add fish in one layer and sauté until lightly browned, about 3 minutes. Turn. Add remaining 1 tablespoon oil. Sauté for 3 minutes.
5. Transfer equal portions to larger compartments of your own TV dinner pans (page 209). Fill smaller compartments with Creamy Mashed Potatoes and Colorful Mixed Vegetables (recipes follow). When ready to serve, garnish with lemon wedges. Serve with My Real Mayonnaise on the side, if desired.

YIELD: Serves 4

NOTES: Any firm-fleshed thinly sliced fish, such as sea bass or halibut, may be substituted for flounder.

If fillets don't fit your skillet in one layer without crowding, cook in 2 batches, using a total of 1 tablespoon oil for each batch.

* To CONVERT into an even more healthful recipe, reduce fat content by substituting Light Mayonnaise (page 182) for My Real Mayonnaise.

*K CREAMY MASHED POTATOES

1 pound baking potatoes, peeled, cut
    into 1-inch cubes
4 teaspoons sweet butter/margarine
    blend
¼ teaspoon each dried dillweed and
    mild paprika

Pinch salt
2 tablespoons cream
¼ cup plain yogurt
¼ cup finely chopped onion or scallion
4 tablespoons finely grated sharp
    cheddar cheese

1. In 1½-quart heavy-bottomed saucepan, cook potatoes in rapidly boiling water until firm-tender, 8 to 10 minutes. Drain well in strainer or colander. Wipe out saucepan. Return potatoes to pan. Cook over medium-high heat, shaking potatoes around pan for about 15 seconds to dry out any excess moisture. Remove from heat.
2. Add 2 teaspoons butter/margarine blend, dill, paprika, and salt. Mash until smooth. Add cream and mash. Stir in yogurt, onion or scallion, and 3 tablespoons cheese. Let cool.
3. Pile into side dishes, mounding on top. Sprinkle with remaining 1 tablespoon grated cheese. Dot with remaining 2 teaspoons butter/margarine blend.

YIELD: Serves 4

* To CONVERT into an even more healthful recipe, reduce fat by substituting milk for cream, and reducing cheddar cheese by half, reserving 1 tablespoon for topping (step 3).

K COLORFUL MIXED VEGETABLES

½ pound green beans, ends trimmed,
    cut into ½-inch pieces
3 medium carrots, peeled, cut into
    ¼-inch dice
4 teaspoons sweet butter/margarine
    blend

⅛ teaspoon each salt, ground
    cinnamon, and freshly grated
    nutmeg
1 teaspoon apple cider vinegar

1. Steam vegetables until firm-tender, about 8 minutes.
2. Melt 2 teaspoons butter/margarine blend in saucepan. Remove from heat. Stir in salt and spices. Add vegetables, gently shaking around pan. Sprinkle with vinegar and stir. Let cool.
3. Fill side dishes, pouring any remaining liquid over vegetables. Dot with reserved 2 teaspoons butter/margarine blend.

YIELD: Serves 4

(34B) *Chicken Dinner*

(Chicken with Peppers, Brown Rice with Mushrooms, Steamed Peas)

CHICKEN WITH PEPPERS

1¼ *pounds skinned and boned chicken*
  breasts, cut into ½-inch strips
2 *teaspoons fresh lemon juice*
4 *tablespoons cornstarch*
1 *teaspoon each ground ginger and*
  dried rosemary leaves, crushed
⅛ *teaspoon salt*
1 *tablespoon Italian olive oil*
1 *tablespoon minced garlic*

1 *medium sweet red pepper, seeded*
  and julienned
1 *teaspoon balsamic vinegar*
⅓ *cup unsweetened pineapple juice*
⅓ *cup My "Canned" Chicken Broth*
  (page 178) or broth made with
  low-sodium vegetable seasoning
¼ *teaspoon ground coriander*
2 *tablespoons minced fresh parsley*

1. Wash and dry chicken thoroughly. Place in bowl. Sprinkle and rub all over with lemon juice. Marinate for 10 minutes.
2. Combine 3 tablespoons cornstarch with ginger, rosemary, and salt. Sprinkle over chicken, rubbing and turning with fingers to coat evenly.
3. Heat oil over medium-high heat in well-seasoned iron or nonstick skillet until hot. Add garlic and red pepper. Sauté for 1 minute. Spread across skillet. Lay chicken on mixture, spreading out in one layer. Cook without stirring for 2 minutes. Turn. Cook for 2 minutes. Add vinegar. Stir and cook for 30 seconds.
4. Measure out 2 tablespoons pineapple juice. Combine in cup with remaining 1 tablespoon cornstarch, stirring until smooth. Set aside.
5. Pour remaining juice and broth around sides of skillet. When bubbly, sprinkle in coriander. Stir and cook for 1 minute. With slotted spoon, transfer equal portions to sides of large plates.
6. While stirring, dribble in cornstarch mixture until thickened. Spoon over chicken. Sprinkle with parsley.
7. Transfer equal portions to larger compartments of your own TV dinner pans (page 209). Fill smaller compartments with Brown Rice with Mushrooms and Steamed Peas (recipes follow).

YIELD: Serves 4

K   BROWN RICE WITH MUSHROOMS

⅔ *cup brown rice*
½ *cup unsweetened pineapple juice*
½ *cup My "Canned" Chicken Broth*
    (page 178) or broth made with
    low-sodium vegetable seasoning
1 *cup water*
1 *teaspoon minced dried onion*
⅛ *teaspoon salt*

2 *tablespoons minced fresh parsley or*
    dill or a combination of both
¼ *pound fresh mushrooms, ends*
    trimmed, rinsed, dried, and
    coarsely chopped
2 *teaspoons sweet butter/margarine*
    blend

1. Soak rice in water to cover for 3 hours. Drain.
2. In heavy-bottomed saucepan, combine drained rice, pineapple juice, Chicken Broth, and water. Bring to boil. Add onion, salt, and 1 tablespoon parsley or dill. Reduce heat to simmer, cover, and cook for 20 minutes.
3. Add mushrooms. Re-cover and simmer for 10 minutes, stirring from time to time. All liquid will be absorbed. Stir. Re-cover and let stand for another 10 minutes. Fluff up with fork.
4. Fill side dishes, mounding on top. Sprinkle with remaining parsley or dill. Dot with butter/margarine blend.

YIELD: Serves 4

K   STEAMED PEAS

1 *pound fresh peas, shelled*
4 *teaspoons sweet butter/margarine*
    blend
½ *teaspoon fresh lemon juice*

½ *teaspoon honey*
⅛ *teaspoon salt*
½ *teaspoon dried tarragon leaves,*
    crumbled

1. Steam peas until almost tender (color should remain bright green).
2. Melt 2 teaspoons butter/margarine blend in saucepan. Remove from heat. Stir in lemon juice, honey, and salt. Add peas and gently shake around pan. Sprinkle with tarragon and shake again. Let cool.
3. Fill side dishes, pouring any remaining liquid over peas. Dot with remaining 2 teaspoons butter/margarine blend.

YIELD: Serves 4

(34C) *Mexican Dinner*

(Mexican Meatballs, Pinto Beans, Crunchy Broccoli, and Super Salsa)

MEXICAN MEATBALLS

Meat:

½ pound each lean beef and pork
2 medium onions
1 small rib celery
3 large cloves garlic
¼ cup tightly packed fresh parsley
 florets
2 tablespoons tomato puree
2 tablespoons apple cider vinegar
½ teaspoon each ground cumin
 and dried oregano leaves
¼ cup regular wheat germ
¼ teaspoon salt
⅛ teaspoon black pepper

Sauce:

2 cloves garlic
2 medium onions
2 tablespoons Italian olive oil
2 tablespoons apple cider vinegar
½ cup tomato puree, preferably
 without salt
1 cup canned crushed tomatoes
1 teaspoon each ground cumin
 and dried oregano leaves
1 4-ounce can mild or spicy green
 chili peppers, chopped
⅛ to ¼ teaspoon black pepper
 Minced fresh coriander

1. Using a food processor fitted with a steel blade, cut meats into chunks. Place in workbowl and process for 10 seconds.
2. Cut onions and celery into chunks; halve each garlic clove. Add to workbowl. Process on/off twice. Add remaining meat ingredients and process until well chopped and combined. With moistened hands, shape into 20 balls, allowing about 1 tablespoon of mixture for each ball.
3. For the sauce, cut up garlic and onions as in step 2. Place in workbowl and process on/off until coarsely chopped. Set aside.
4. Heat oil over medium-high heat in a well-seasoned iron skillet until hot. Add meatballs and brown all over. Add chopped garlic and onion and lightly brown, stirring constantly.
5. Spoon vinegar around sides of skillet. Cook for 30 seconds. Stir in tomato puree and crushed tomatoes. Add cumin, oregano, chili peppers, and black pepper. Bring to simmering point, gently turning meatballs to coat. Cover and simmer for 15 minutes, spooning meat with sauce from time to time. Remove from heat. Let stand, covered, for 30 minutes. Chill until sauce congeals.
6. Arrange 5 balls on sides of each large plate. Spoon with equal amount of sauce. Sprinkle with fresh coriander.
7. Transfer equal portions to larger compartments of your own TV dinner pans (page 209). Fill smaller compartments with Pinto Beans and Crunchy Broccoli (recipes follow). Serve Super Salsa on the side.

YIELD: Serves 4

K PINTO BEANS

1 cup pinto beans, picked over and
    soaked for at least 4 hours
3½ cups My "Canned" Chicken Broth
    (page 178) or broth made with
    low-sodium vegetable seasoning
½ teaspoon each ground cumin and
    ginger

1 tablespoon Italian olive oil
1 tablespoon minced garlic
⅔ cup coarsely chopped onion
1 tablespoon apple cider vinegar
¼ teaspoon salt
    Chopped sweet red pepper, or
    jarred chopped pimentos, drained

1. Drain beans. Place in heavy-bottomed saucepan or kettle. Add balance of ingredients except red pepper. Bring to boil. Reduce heat to simmering. Cover and simmer until tender, about 1 hour. Drain. Let cool.
2. Fill side dishes. Sprinkle with sweet red pepper or garnish with pimentos.

YIELD: Serves 4 to 5

VARIATION: Before draining at end of step 1, with slotted spoon measure out ⅓ cup beans. Place in workbowl of food processor fitted with steel blade. Add 1 tablespoon cooking liquid. Puree until smooth. Drain remaining beans. Combine puree with whole beans. Continue with step 2.

K CRUNCHY BROCCOLI

3 loosely packed cups fresh broccoli
    florets
4 teaspoons sweet butter/margarine
    blend
1 teaspoon fresh lemon juice

⅛ teaspoon each salt and freshly grated
    nutmeg
1 tablespoon finely grated orange rind,
    preferably from navel orange

1. Steam broccoli for 3 minutes (it will be undercooked and bright green).
2. Melt 2 teaspoons butter/margarine blend in saucepan. Remove from heat. Stir in balance of ingredients. Add broccoli and gently shake around pan. Let cool.
3. Fill side dishes, pouring any remaining liquid over broccoli. Dot with remaining butter/margarine blend.

YIELD: Serves 4 to 5

SUPER SALSA

2 medium carrots, peeled	1 teaspoon dried oregano leaves
2 large onions	¼ to ½ teaspoon salt
1 sweet red or green pepper, seeded	½ teaspoon ground cumin
2 ribs celery	2 pounds ripe fresh tomatoes, cored, peeled, and chopped
3 large cloves garlic	½ cup apple cider vinegar
¼ cup rinsed and tightly packed fresh coriander leaves	¼ cup tomato paste
2 tablespoons Italian olive oil	⅛ teaspoon cayenne or black pepper

1. Cut carrot, onion, pepper, and celery into uniform-size chunks; halve each garlic clove.
2. Fit food processor with steel blade. Place vegetable chunks in workbowl, and process on/off 3 times. Add garlic and coriander. Process on/off until vegetables are chopped into ⅛-inch pieces.
3. Heat oil in large nonstick skillet until hot. Add chopped ingredients. Sprinkle with oregano, salt, and cumin. Stir and sauté over medium heat until mixture is wilted but not brown.
4. In bowl, combine and stir tomatoes, vinegar, and tomato paste. Add to skillet. Bring to simmering point. Cover and simmer for 15 minutes. Let cool. Stir in red or black pepper. Store in refrigerator in tightly closed jar. Serve well chilled.

YIELD: 1 quart; serving size = ½ cup

VARIATION: Just before serving, stir in 2 tablespoons dairy sour cream for each cup of well-chilled salsa.*

* To CONVERT into an even more healthful variation, reduce fat content by using low-fat plain yogurt in place of sour cream.

(35)* COPYCAT CHICKEN McNUGGETS

1 egg	¼ teaspoon each ground ginger and curry powder
2 tablespoons unsweetened apple juice	
2 tablespoons cream	1¼ pounds boned and skinned thick chicken breasts
¼ teaspoon salt	
⅓ cup fine bread crumbs, preferably homemade (see Note)	2 tablespoons oil
	4 large cloves garlic, quartered
2 tablespoons unbleached flour	½ lemon
¾ teaspoon each dried rosemary leaves, crushed, and onion powder	

1. In bowl, combine and blend egg, apple juice, and cream. In another bowl, place salt, bread crumbs, flour, rosemary, and spices, stirring to combine. Spread mixture across flat plate.
2. Wash and dry chicken thoroughly. Cut into 1-inch chunks. Drop into egg mixture. Drain each piece; then dip into crumb mixture, rolling to evenly coat. Place plate in freezer, uncovered, for 10 minutes to set.
3. Sauté in 2 batches. Heat 1 tablespoon oil in large well-seasoned iron skillet until hot but not smoking. Add half of garlic and cook for 1 minute, stirring continually. With slotted spoon, remove and discard garlic. Add half of chicken. Cook until lightly browned on both sides, rolling when necessary to brown all areas (total cooking time 6 minutes). Transfer to warm oven or to plate over simmering water while second batch is cooked (do not cover).
4. To prepare second batch, add remaining tablespoon of oil to skillet (it will heat rapidly). Sauté remaining garlic and continue to cook as in step 3. Squeeze lemon juice over chicken and serve immediately.

YIELD: Serves 4

NOTE: Make your own bread crumbs. It's easy. Use 3 to 4 slices Italian or French bread, or 3 thick slices Wonder-Ful Bread (page 186). Cut into ½-inch cubes. Spread on cookie sheet and bake in preheated 425°F. oven for 8 to 10 minutes, turning once with spatula. Let cool. Transfer to food blender and blend on high speed for 1 minute. Use immediately, or pour into jar, tightly close, and store in refrigerator (up to 2 weeks).

* To CONVERT into an even more healthful recipe, reduce fat content by substituting equal amount milk for cream.

(36)*K "FRIED" CHICKEN

1 tablespoon fresh lemon juice
2 tablespoons frozen orange juice
    concentrate
2 tablespoons evaporated milk
1 tablespoon water
1 3-pound broiling chicken, skinned,
    wing tips removed, cut into
    eighths

½ cup My Shake and Bake-Alike (page
    175)
2 tablespoons oil
1 tablespoon sweet butter/margarine
    blend, cut into small pieces
⅓ cup finely grated sharp cheddar
    cheese

1. In large bowl, combine first 4 ingredients. Blend with fork.
2. Pierce chicken all over with sharp-pronged fork. Add to bowl, turning to coat. Cover and let stand for 1 hour at room temperature. Drain each piece of chicken; then lay on double sheet of paper toweling and gently blot (do not rub), so that chicken is still moist.

3. Sprinkle half of Shake and Bake-Alike across large flat plate. Lay chicken pieces atop mixture, pressing to adhere. Sprinkle with remaining mix, pressing into chicken all over. Refrigerate, uncovered, for 30 minutes or longer.
4. Preheat oven to 425°F. Spread oil over shallow baking pan large enough to hold chicken in one layer. Place pan in oven for 7 minutes. Reduce heat to 400°F. Immediately arrange chicken in pan in one layer. Dot with shortening. Bake for 20 minutes. Carefully turn with spatula, scooping up so that browned pieces remain on chicken. Return to oven and bake for 10 minutes more. Sprinkle with cheese and bake for another 10 to 15 minutes, or until browned and fork-tender.

YIELD: Serves 4 to 5

VARIATION: Add 1 teaspoon dried sage to My Shake and Bake-Alike (step 3).

NOTE: Chicken is delicious served cold. If you're planning to serve it cold, add ¼ teaspoon salt to Shake and Bake-Alike before coating chicken.

* To CONVERT into an even more healthful recipe, reduce fat content by substituting equal amount part-skim mozzarella cheese, or 2 tablespoons freshly grated Parmesan cheese, for cheddar cheese.

(37) *   CHICKEN WITH CHEESE

1¼ pounds skinned and boned thick
  chicken breasts
1 teaspoon dried sage leaves
⅛ teaspoon salt
¼ teaspoon each ground cinnamon,
  curry, and coriander
2 tablespoons sweet butter/margarine
  blend
¼ cup minced shallots
2 teaspoons minced garlic

⅓ cup My "Canned" Chicken Broth
  (page 178) or broth made with
  low-sodium vegetable seasoning
1 teaspoon salt-reduced soy sauce
1 teaspoon fresh lemon juice
⅓ cup dairy sour cream
3 tablespoons finely grated sharp
  cheddar cheese
2 tablespoons minced fresh parsley

1. Wash and dry chicken thoroughly. Prick all over with sharp-pronged fork.
2. In cup, combine and blend sage, salt, and spices. Sprinkle and rub over chicken.
3. Heat butter/margarine blend over medium heat in well-seasoned iron skillet until moderately hot. Add shallots and garlic. Sauté for 2 minutes without browning. Add chicken, turning to coat. Cook for 30 seconds on each side.
4. Combine Chicken Broth with soy sauce. Pour around sides of skillet. Bring to slow boil, turning chicken twice to coat.

5. Preheat oven to 375°F. Cover skillet loosely with aluminum foil. Bake for 15 minutes.
6. Drain liquid into cup. Whisk in lemon juice and sour cream. Spoon mixture over chicken. Sprinkle chicken with cheese and parsley. Place skillet under broiler at low level and broil until cheese melts to a golden brown. Serve immediately.

YIELD: Serves 4

* To CONVERT into an even more healthful recipe, reduce fat content by substituting equal amount of low-fat plain yogurt for dairy sour cream, and part-skim mozzarella cheese for cheddar cheese.

(38) MEAT LOAF "MUFFINS"

1 cup My Frozen Vegetable Mix (page 173)
½ cup My "Canned" Chicken Broth (page 178) or broth made with low-sodium vegetable seasoning
3 tablespoons tomato paste
½ teaspoon finely chopped lemon rind
1 tablespoon balsamic vinegar
½ pound each lean ground beef and veal

3 tablespoons freshly grated Parmesan cheese
½ cup toasted fine bread crumbs, preferably homemade (page 217)
¼ teaspoon each freshly grated nutmeg, salt, and ground allspice
1 teaspoon dried basil leaves, crumbled
1 egg, lightly beaten

1. In heavy-bottomed saucepan, combine Vegetable Mix, broth, tomato paste, and lemon rind. Bring to boil, breaking up Vegetable Mix with spoon as mixture heats. Stir well. Reduce heat to slow boil, and cook, uncovered, until most of liquid evaporates, stirring from time to time. Add vinegar. Stir and cook for 1 minute. Let cool.
2. In bowl, combine remaining ingredients, blending well. Add cooled vegetable mixture, and blend again.
3. Preheat oven to 425°F. Using sweet butter/margarine blend, well-grease 3-inch muffin pans. Divide meat into 8 equal pieces, shaping each piece into smooth ball. Drop each ball into muffin pans, pressing gently on top with hands. Cover loosely with aluminum foil. Bake for 15 minutes. Reduce heat to 400°F. and bake for 15 minutes. Remove from oven. Let stand for 5 minutes. Run blunt knife around sides of pans. Remove muffins, and serve.

YIELD: 8 muffins

VARIATIONS: Spread with cheese: After muffins have baked a total of 20 minutes, top each muffin with ¼-inch slices of mozzarella cheese. Sprinkle with paprika. Return to oven and bake for 10 minutes.

Spread with potato "icing": Prepare mashed potatoes by cooking ¾ pound peeled and diced potatoes until tender. Drain. Beat until fluffy with 1 tablespoon sweet butter/margarine blend, 1 tablespoon plain yogurt, 1½ teaspoons egg yolk, and salt and black pepper to taste. After muffins have baked for 25 minutes, remove pan from oven and let stand for 5 minutes. Carefully remove muffins and place on lightly greased baking pan. Spread tops with thick layer of mashed potatoes. Striate with fork. Brush lightly with melted butter/margarine blend. Brown briefly under medium heat in broiler.

Make a meat loaf: Shape meat into an 8″ x 4″ loaf. Place in lightly oiled baking pan. Preheat oven to 400°F. Cover loosely with aluminum foil. Bake for 40 minutes. Let stand, partially covered, for 5 minutes before slicing. Loaf yields eight 1-inch slices.

(39)*K   LASAGNA

1½ teaspoons oil
¼ teaspoon salt
½ pound lasagna noodles
    Sweet butter/margarine blend
4½ cups Spaghetti Sauce (page 194)
½ pound mozzarella cheese, thinly
    sliced

1 15-ounce container ricotta cheese,
    at room temperature
½ cup freshly grated Parmesan cheese
¼ cup finely grated sharp cheddar
    cheese
¼ cup minced fresh basil leaves (see
    Note)

1. To cook noodles, bring large pot of water to boil. Add 1 teaspoon oil and salt. Carefully ease 2 to 3 noodles at a time into water. Boil for 8 to 10 minutes, until firm-tender. Pour into colander and drain. Rinse under cold running water and drain well.
2. Grease a 7″ x 9″ ovenproof dish with butter/margarine blend. Spoon a thin layer of Spaghetti Sauce over dish. Arrange one-third of noodles in one layer over sauce. Spread one-third of sauce over noodles. Lay one-third of mozzarella cheese over sauce. Cover with one-third of ricotta cheese, spreading out with knife. Sprinkle with one-third each of Parmesan, cheddar cheese, and minced basil. Repeat layering sequence twice more.
3. Preheat oven to 375°F. Cover dish with sheet of aluminum foil. Bake for 20 minutes. Reduce heat to 350°F. Uncover, and bake for 20 to 25 minutes, or until bubbly and hot. Cut and serve at once.

Yield: Serves 8 to 10

Variation: For meatless lasagna, substitute Pizza Sauce (page 194) for Spaghetti Sauce.

Note: Fresh herbs enhance flavor. If fresh basil isn't available, substitute minced fresh rosemary, dill, or parsley.

* To convert into an even more healthful recipe, reduce fat content by using part-skim ricotta and mozzarella cheese, and eliminating cheddar cheese.

(40)K   RICE MIX

½ cup each brown rice and wild rice
1 cup unsweetened apple juice
1 cup water
1 cup My "Canned" Chicken Broth (page 178) or broth made with low-sodium vegetable seasoning

1 teaspoon My Spicy Mix (page 177)
⅛ teaspoon salt

1. Combine and stir all ingredients in 1½- to 2-quart heavy-bottomed saucepan. Soak for 2 hours.
2. Bring to boil. Stir vigorously. Reduce heat, cover, and simmer, stirring twice at equal intervals, until all liquid is absorbed (40 to 50 minutes). Mixture will be tender and moist.

Yield: About 2¾ cups; serves 5

(41)K   TOP-OF-THE-STOVE STUFFING

3 tablespoons plus 1 teaspoon My Seasoning Mix (page 176)
1¼ cups water or My "Canned" Chicken Broth (page 178)
¼ cup sweet butter/margarine blend

3 cups ½-inch cubed and toasted French or Italian bread or a combination of French or Italian bread and whole-wheat bread

1. In 1½- to 2-quart heavy-bottomed saucepan, combine Seasoning Mix, water or broth, and butter/margarine blend. Bring to boil. Reduce heat to simmering. Cover and simmer for 3 minutes.
2. Stir in bread cubes. Fluff up with fork. Cover and let stand for 3 minutes.

Yield: About 3 cups; serves 5

Serving suggestion: Serve as side dish along with meat, fish, or poultry instead of potatoes.

Variations: In step 2, add ⅓ cup chopped unsweetened canned chestnuts or roasted fresh chestnuts and/or ¼ cup chopped soaked dried apricots (without added preservatives).

Add 2 chopped and sautéed chicken livers to stuffing after bread has been added in step 2.

Note: For a moister stuffing, increase water or broth by 2 tablespoons; for a drier stuffing, decrease water or broth by 2 tablespoons.

(42)*K "POUCH-TYPE" BROCCOLI IN ORANGE SAUCE

1 *bunch broccoli (about 1½ pounds)*
2 *tablespoons sweet butter/margarine*
  blend
1 *tablespoon unbleached flour*
1 *tablespoon frozen orange juice*
  concentrate
⅔ *cup evaporated milk*

2 *tablespoons finely grated sharp*
  cheddar cheese
¼ *teaspoon freshly grated nutmeg*
⅛ *teaspoon each salt and black pepper*
¼ *teaspoon curry powder*
  Minced fresh parsley

1. Cut broccoli 2 to 3 inches down from florets. To promote tenderness and reduce the bitterness that usually accompanies broccoli, peel off the skin from stems. Steam.
2. Melt shortening over low heat in heavy-bottomed pot (preferably with enamel coating). Add flour and stir with wooden spoon for 1 minute.
3. Combine orange juice with milk. Add slowly to pot and blend with whisk until smooth. Whisk in cheese, nutmeg, salt, pepper, and curry powder. Cook while stirring for 2 minutes.
4. Arrange steamed broccoli on serving plate. Spoon with sauce, sprinkle with parsley, and serve immediately.

Yield: Entire dish serves 4; sauce alone, ¾ cup

Serving suggestions: Sauce is delicious served over any steamed vegetable or steamed white-fleshed fish. If served over fish, add a sprinkling of fresh lemon juice just before serving.

* To convert into an even more healthful recipe, reduce fat content by substituting freshly grated Parmesan cheese for cheddar cheese, and fresh skim milk instead of evaporated milk.

(43)*K BARBECUE SAUCE

1 *cup unsweetened apple juice*
¼ *cup minced shallots or onion*
2 *teaspoons dark brown sugar*
¼ *teaspoon each dry mustard, chili con*
  carne seasoning, and
  Worcestershire sauce

¼ *teaspoon salt*
¼ *cup tomato puree or Ketchup De-Lite*
  (page 199)
1 *tablespoon balsamic vinegar*
2 *tablespoons minced fresh parsley*

1. Combine juice, shallots or onion, sugar, and seasonings in small heavy-bottomed saucepan. Bring to boil. Reduce heat and simmer for 2 minutes. Remove from heat and let cool.
2. Stir in tomato puree or Ketchup De-Lite, vinegar, and parsley. Store in tightly closed glass container in refrigerator for up to 10 days.

YIELD: About 1½ cups, serving size = up to 3 tablespoons

SERVING SUGGESTION: Use as basting sauce or marinade for meat or chicken.

* To CONVERT into an even more healthful recipe, substitute 1 tablespoon honey for 2 teaspoons brown sugar.

(44)* VEGETABLE SLAW

1 pound zucchini, well scrubbed	2 tablespoons apple cider vinegar
3 large slender carrots, peeled	3 tablespoons each My Real
1 small sweet green or red pepper,	Mayonnaise (page 180) and dairy
seeded	sour cream
1 small onion	¼ teaspoon each mild paprika and salt
1 teaspoon sugar	¼ cup dark raisins

1. Using food processor fitted with grating blade, grate zucchini and carrots. Turn into large bowl. There should be about 5¾ loosely packed cups.
2. Fit processor with steel blade. Cut pepper and onion into uniform chunks. Place in workbowl of processor and coarsely chop. Add to zucchini and carrots, stirring to combine.
3. In small bowl, whisk sugar with vinegar until smooth. Then whisk in mayonnaise, sour cream, paprika, and salt. Pour over vegetables, tossing gently to coat. Stir in raisins.
4. Refrigerate, covered, for at least 1 hour, stirring once midway.

YIELD: 1 loosely packed quart; serves 6 to 8

* To CONVERT into an even more healthful recipe, use honey instead of sugar; and to reduce fat content, substitute Light Mayonnaise (page 182) for Real Mayonnaise, and low-fat plain yogurt for dairy sour cream.

(45)* CRANAPPLE SAUCE

1 cup My Frozen Vegetable Mix (page
   173)
½ cup apple cider vinegar
3 medium crisp sweet apples, such as
   Washington State, peeled, cored,
   and coarsely chopped
½ cup dark raisins
⅔ cup fresh cranberries, picked over
   and well rinsed

⅛ teaspoon ground allspice
½ teaspoon ground ginger
½ lime, seeded and cubed
1 tablespoon frozen orange juice
   concentrate
2 tablespoons each sugar and honey

1. Combine all ingredients except honey in a 2-quart stainless-steel pot or
   waterless cooker. Bring to boil. Reduce heat to simmering. Cover and simmer for 1¾ hours, stirring from time to time. Uncover, and simmer for 15
   minutes, stirring often. Remove from heat, partially cover, and let stand for
   30 minutes. Stir in honey.
2. For fully developed flavor, refrigerate in tightly closed jar overnight. Sauce
   will keep for 10 days in refrigerator.

YIELD: About 2¾ cups; serving size = ¼ cup

* To CONVERT into an even more healthful recipe, eliminate sugar, increase
honey to 3 tablespoons, and cut back to ¼ lime. Lime is a healthful food, but
less of it requires less sweetening.

(46)* DESSERT TOPPING

¾ cup plain yogurt
3 tablespoons cream
¼ teaspoon ground cinnamon
⅛ teaspoon freshly grated nutmeg

1 tablespoon unsweetened shredded
   coconut
1½ teaspoons honey

Combine all ingredients in small bowl. Gently fold in ingredients (do not
beat). Let stand for 10 minutes before serving. Serve chilled.

YIELD: 1 cup, serving size = up to ¼ cup

SERVING SUGGESTION: Great with pancakes, over fruit, or mixed with My Fruit
Butter (page 178).

* To CONVERT into an even more healthful recipe, substitute milk for cream
(less fat) and 2 teaspoons date powder for coconut (to eliminate the saturated
fat in the coconut while maintaining sweetness).

(47)* HAPPY BIRTHDAY CAKE

Imagine—a rich, sweet-tasting, creamy-iced birthday cake that uses less than 1 teaspoon sugar per serving. Most store-bought and homemade cakes use 16 teaspoons or more per serving.

The icing is a clone of dark, chocolate fudge buttercream, but it has none of the health-drawbacks of its conventional counterpart. Chocolate is replaced by carob, a naturally sweet plant product which tastes like chocolate in this confection; and the butter content is reduced. Use the icing also for a low-sugar, healthful chocolate-brown smooth fudge sauce over ice cream, custard, fruit or plain cake.

Serve this cake unadorned by icing *any* day for a scrumptious treat.

Cake:

½ cup sweet butter/margarine blend, plus enough to grease pans
2 tablespoons corn oil
½ cup My Fruit Butter (page 178)
1 cup mashed ripe bananas (2 medium bananas)
2 teaspoons pure vanilla extract
4 eggs, separated
3¾ cups My Muffin and Cake Mix (page 172)
1 teaspoon baking soda
1 teaspoon ground ginger
1½ cups milk
¼ cup finely chopped walnuts
¼ cup date powder
1 teaspoon ground cinnamon
⅛ teaspoon cream of tartar

Fudge Icing:

1½ cups unsweetened carob chips (available in health-food stores)
¾ teaspoon ground cinnamon
¼ teaspoon salt
6 tablespoons honey
4½ teaspoons sugar
1 2-inch piece vanilla bean, split
3 teaspoons grain coffee
3 egg yolks
¾ cup evaporated milk
1⅛ cups sweet butter/margarine blend

Decoration:

Shredded unsweetened coconut
Blanched almond halves or plastic Happy Birthday decoration

1. Place first 5 ingredients in large bowl of mixing machine. Beat on medium speed for 1 minute, then on high speed until light and fluffy, scraping down sides of bowl when necessary.
2. Reduce speed to medium. Add egg yolks. Beat for 1 minute. Scrape down sides of bowl.
3. Combine Muffin and Cake Mix with baking soda and ginger. Add to batter alternately with milk, ½ cup at a time. Stop machine. Scrape down sides.
4. In cup, combine walnuts, date powder, and cinnamon. Sprinkle over batter. With wooden spoon, stir without blending into batter, using 5 or 6 broad strokes.

5. Beat egg whites until foamy. Sprinkle in cream of tartar. Beat until stiff but not dry peaks form. Fold one-third into batter; fold in balance, using as few strokes as possible.
6. Preheat oven to 350°F. Pour batter into two round removable-bottomed 8-inch layer pans. Bake for 45 minutes, or until toothpick inserted into center comes out clean. (Don't be concerned if cakes crack slightly in centers.)
7. Place on rack. Let cool for 5 minutes. With blunt knife, loosen around sides. Remove loose bottom from sides with cake and place on rack. Let cakes cool for 15 minutes. Using large spatula, ease cakes off loose bottom onto rack. Let cool completely before icing.
8. To prepare icing, use a double boiler. Place first 7 ingredients in top part. Cook while stirring over simmering water for 5 minutes. Mixture will be thick and smooth. In bowl, beat egg yolks with fork. Stir in milk and blend. Pour into carob mixture. Stir and cook until thick and smooth (about 5 minutes). Let cool. Remove vanilla bean, pressing out juices.
9. Place shortening in large mixing bowl. Beat on high speed until smooth. Beat in cooled carob mixture, a little at a time, until well blended. Icing will become thin. Chill until spreadable, about 30 minutes.
10. To assemble, using serrated knife, slice each layer horizontally in half. Place bottom of one layer on sheet of waxed paper on firm surface. Spread with a fifth of icing. Cover with cake layer. Continue to ice between layers, on top and around sides of cake in an attractive pattern. Sprinkle coconut around outer edge of iced top layer. Chill until icing is firm to the touch.
11. Write, using almonds, "Happy Birthday," in the center of the cake, pressing each nut (but not too forcefully) into the icing, or use plastic decoration. Let stand at room temperature for 1 hour before serving.

YIELD: 16 or more servings

FUDGE ICING VARIATION: For a pourable consistency for serving over plain cake, muffins, ice cream, or fruit increase evaporated milk to 1¼ cups. Use 1 cup in step 8. Stir in 2 tablespoons sweet butter/margarine blend at end of step 8. Stir in as much of the remaining ¼ cup milk as necessary to thin to desired consistency.

* To CONVERT into an even more healthful recipe, use converted Muffin and Cake Mix. For decoration around edges of top layer, substitute chopped walnuts for coconut, which is high in saturated fat.

(48)* PLUM CAKE OR APPLE CAKE

Cake Base:

⅓ cup sweet butter/margarine
blend
¼ cup My Fruit Butter (page
178)
1 tablespoon frozen orange juice
concentrate

½ teaspoon pure vanilla extract
2 eggs
2½ cups My Muffin and Cake
Mix (page 172)
Scant cup milk or water or a mixture
of both

Plum Streusel Topping:

14 to 16 small purple plums, pitted and
quartered
½ teaspoon finely chopped lemon
rind
2 tablespoons unbleached flour
2 tablespoons date powder
½ teaspoon ground cinnamon

¼ teaspoon freshly grated
nutmeg
1 tablespoon sweet butter/
margarine blend
1 tablespoon honey dissolved in
1 tablespoon water

Apple Streusel Topping:

1 tablespoon fresh lemon juice
4 medium Golden Delicious
apples, peeled and cored
2 tablespoons unbleached flour
3 tablespoons date powder
1 teaspoon ground cinnamon

¼ teaspoon freshly ground
nutmeg or cardamom
2 tablespoons sweet butter/
margarine blend
1 tablespoon honey dissolved in
1 tablespoon water

1. To prepare cake base, in mixing bowl, combine first 4 ingredients. Using mixing machine, beat on medium speed until mixture is well blended, scraping down sides with rubber spatula once.
2. With machine going, add eggs, one at a time, and beat until combined. Spoon in Muffin and Cake Mix alternately with milk and blend.
3. Grease a 9-inch square pan and preheat oven to 350°F. Spread batter in pan.

To complete plum cake

4. Arrange plums side by side, cut edges down, on top of batter in a neat pattern. Press gently into batter.
5. Place lemon rind, flour, date powder, and spices in small bowl. Using pastry blender or 2 knives, cut shortening into dry ingredients to make a crumbly mixture. Sprinkle over plums. Bake for 55 to 60 minutes, or until browned edges of cake come way from sides of pan. Place on rack. Drizzle with honey/water mixture and let cool in pan for 30 minutes.

To complete apple cake

6. Pour lemon juice into bowl. Cut apples into ⅜-inch slices and drop slices into bowl as they're cut, turning to coat. Arrange apple slices side by side on top of cake base in a neat pattern. Press gently into batter.
7. Place flour, date powder, and spices in small bowl. Using pastry blender or 2 knives, cut shortening into dry ingredients to make a crumbly mixture. Sprinkle over apples. Bake for 55 to 60 minutes, or until browned edges of cake come away from sides of pan. Place on rack. Drizzle with honey/water mixture and let cool in pan for 30 minutes.
8. Cut plum or apple cake into 16 serving pieces. Serve slightly warm or at room temperature.

YIELD: 16 squares of each cake

NOTES: If plums or apples are very tart, increase honey to 2 tablespoons, and dissolve in 1 tablespoon water. Drizzle over cake in steps 5 and 7.

Cakes are delicious next day if wrapped in aluminum foil, refrigerated, and reheated briefly. Freeze leftovers by wrapping each square in aluminum foil and placing in plastic bags; tightly seal. A frozen square, placed in your child's lunchbox in the morning, will be defrosted and ready to enjoy by lunchtime.

* To CONVERT into an even more healthful recipe, use converted Muffin and Cake Mix in cake base.

(49) * BLUEBERRY MOUSSE

1 6-ounce can evaporated milk
⅓ cup whipping cream
2 teaspoons unflavored gelatin
¼ teaspoon freshly grated nutmeg

½ cup cold Blueberry Sauce (page 235)
1 tablespoon black cherry concentrate
 (available in health-food stores)

1. Pour milk into mixing bowl. Stand bowl in freezer compartment of refrigerator in direct contact with metal. Place whipping utensil in freezer as well. Freeze milk until almost solid.
2. When milk is almost frozen, pour ¼ cup cream into small heavy-bottomed saucepan (preferably enameled). Sprinkle with gelatin. Let stand for 3 minutes to soften. Place over low heat and cook to simmering point, stirring briefly with wooden spoon until mixture is smooth. Whisk in nutmeg and remaining cream. Let cool briefly without setting. Remove milk from freezer.
3. With mixing machine, at high speed, beat almost-frozen milk for 2 minutes. With machine running, add gelatin mixture, a little at a time, and continue to beat until stiff.

4. In cup, combine Blueberry Sauce with black cherry concentrate. Fold into whipped mixture (do not overfold). Spoon into 6 dessert dishes. Chill until set.

YIELD: Serves 6

VARIATION: Serve as a frozen dessert. Pour contents of bowl in step 4 into large freezer tray. Freeze until almost firm.

* To CONVERT into an even more healthful recipe, reduce fat content by substituting an additional ⅓ cup evaporated milk for whipping cream.

(50) "SUPERMARKET" CAKE

Cake:

1½ cups unbleached flour
½ teaspoon baking soda
1½ teaspoons baking powder
¼ cup sweet butter/margarine blend,
    plus some for pan
2 tablespoons corn oil
½ cup date powder

1 tablespoon honey
1 teaspoon pure vanilla extract
2 eggs
1 cup plain yogurt
½ cup dark raisins or unsweetened
    carob chips

Swirl Topping:

¼ teaspoon freshly grated nutmeg
1 teaspoon ground cinnamon

2 tablespoons date powder
⅓ cup coarsely chopped walnuts

1. Onto large sheet of waxed paper (or into bowl) sift flour, baking soda, and baking powder. Set aside.
2. In large bowl of mixing machine, on high speed, cream shortening, oil, date powder, and honey until well blended and light, scraping down sides of bowl several times. Beat in vanilla and eggs, one at a time. Add yogurt. Beat on medium speed for 30 seconds.
3. Funnel flour-covered waxed paper, and with machine running on low speed, add dry mixture, a little at a time, until just moistened. Stir in raisins or carob chips by hand.
4. Lightly grease a 9-inch loose-bottomed tube pan with shortening. Preheat oven to 350°F. Spoon batter into pan.
5. Prepare swirl topping by combining all ingredients in cup. Sprinkle over batter. With spoon, fold topping into batter in 4 or 5 places (do not mix), smoothing out top.

6. Bake for 45 to 50 minutes. Cake is done when browned and toothpick inserted comes out clean. With blunt knife, loosen around sides of pan. Lift out tube and place on rack. Let cake cool in tube before removing.

YIELD: 10 or more servings

(51) ICED BANANA POPSICLES

4 ripe medium bananas
1½ teaspoons sweet butter/margarine
   blend
2 teaspoons honey
¼ cup unsweetened apple juice
1 1-inch piece vanilla bean, split
3 tablespoons unsweetened carob
   powder

3 tablespoons each unshelled sesame
   seeds, regular wheat germ, and
   chopped walnuts
½ teaspoon ground cinnamon
8 wooden Popsicle sticks

1. Place unpeeled bananas in freezer for 20 minutes.
2. In small heavy-bottomed saucepan, melt butter/margarine blend over low heat. While stirring, dribble in honey. Add apple juice and vanilla bean. Bring to simmering point. Sprinkle in carob, breaking up any lumps. Stir until dissolved. Cook, uncovered, until mixture is satiny smooth and slightly thickened, about 3 minutes. Remove from heat. Let cool to room temperature.
3. In cup, combine sesame seeds, wheat germ, nuts, and cinnamon. Line small baking pan with waxed paper. Sprinkle with half of mixture.
4. Remove bananas from freezer and carefully peel. Cut each banana in half. Insert wooden sticks into bananas lengthwise. Dip each half into carob mixture, gently rolling with fork to coat. Lay atop wheat germ mixture. Sprinkle with balance of wheat germ mixture, turning with fork to evenly coat.
5. Place in freezer. Popsicles are ready to enjoy in 2 hours.

YIELD: 8 Popsicles

(52)K ICE CREAM MILK SHAKE

1 cup ice-cold unsweetened apple
   juice

1 scoop Peach or Black Cherry–Banana
   Ice Cream (page 206 or 207)

1. Combine apple juice and ice cream in food blender. Blend on high speed until smooth and frothy.
2. Pour into tall glass and serve immediately.

YIELD: Serves 1

Recipes for the
New "Bright Cuisine"

The **numbers in parentheses** correspond to titles in the list on pages 154–55, from which you can plan your Bright Cuisine replacements in the Basic All-Family Menu Plan. The **letter K** means the recipe is simple enough for your kids to make under your supervision. Recipes are arranged under *Breakfast*, *Lunch*, and *Dinner*.

Bright Cuisine Dishes
for Breakfast

(53) WHOLE-WHEAT BREAD

1 tablespoon dark honey
¼ cup warm water (105° to 115°F.), plus 1 scant cup water
1 package dry yeast
2½ to 2¾ cups unbleached flour
1½ cups stone-ground whole-wheat flour
1 teaspoon ground coriander
½ teaspoon ground cinnamon
¼ teaspoon salt
¼ cup date powder
2 tablespoons nonfat dry milk solids
¼ cup low-fat plain yogurt
1 tablespoon oil
3 tablespoons frozen apple juice concentrate

1. In tall glass, combine molasses with ¼ cup warm water, stirring to dissolve. Sprinkle in yeast and flour. Stir. Let stand until mixture rises to top of glass, about 7 minutes.
2. Fit food processor with steel blade. In workbowl, combine 2¼ cups unbleached flour, all of whole-wheat flour, spices, salt, date powder, and dry milk. Process on/off 4 times.
3. Add yeast mixture. Process until blended. Add yogurt and oil. Process for 10 seconds.
4. Combine and heat apple juice concentrate and scant cup water until warm (90°F.). With machine running, slowly pour through feed tube. Process

until ball rotates around workbowl 15 to 20 times, using remaining flour, if necessary, to make a nonsticky ball. Transfer to board and knead by hand for 1 minute. Shape into ball.

5. Lightly oil a fairly straight-sided bowl. Drop dough in, turning to coat. Cover with plastic wrap. Let rise at room temperature (70° to 80°F.) until doubled in bulk, about 1½ hours. Punch down. Knead briefly. Cut in half.

6. Shape each half into a ball. Flatten with hands. Using a rolling pin, roll each piece into a rectangle wide enough to fit loaf pan. Tightly roll up, pinching ends. Grease two 7⅜" x 3⅝" x 2¼" pans and 2 sheets of waxed paper. Place dough seam down in pans and cover with waxed paper. Let rise until well above sides of pans, about 1 hour. Preheat oven to 375°F.

7. Bake for 35 to 40 minutes. Remove from pan. Test for doneness by tapping bottom of loaves with knuckles. A hollow sound indicates that bread is done. If bread is not done, return loaves to oven and bake for another 5 minutes. Let cool completely before slicing.

YIELD: 2 loaves

VARIATION: Raisin Whole-Wheat Bread: Add ¼ cup raisins to saucepan in step 4. Heat until very warm (105° to 115°F.). Let mixture cool for 10 minutes. Continue with balance of instructions.

(54) NO-KNEAD RAISIN BREAD

2 tablespoons sweet butter/margarine blend, cut into small pieces
⅓ cup dark raisins
1 cup boiling water
1 package dry yeast
2 cups My Pancake Mix (page 174)
½ cup stone-ground whole-wheat flour
¼ cup buckwheat flour
1 teaspoon plus 1 tablespoon honey
1 teaspoon ground coriander
½ teaspoon salt
1 egg
½ cup thick buttermilk, preferably without salt added, at room temperature
1 teaspoon finely chopped orange rind

1. Place shortening and raisins in small bowl. Pour boiling water over mixture. Let stand until cooled down to very hot (105° to 115°F.).

2. Using mixing machine, in bowl combine yeast, Pancake Mix, whole-wheat flour, 1 teaspoon honey, coriander, and salt. Add hot raisin mixture. Beat on low speed for 2 minutes.

3. In cup, combine 1 tablespoon honey with egg and buttermilk. With mixing machine on low speed, add to bowl and beat for 1 minute. Stop machine; scrape down sides. Add orange rind. Beat on medium speed for 2 minutes. Mixture will be pully and sticky.

4. Grease a 9-inch loaf pan and oil a sheet of waxed paper. Turn batter into pan and cover with waxed paper. Let rise at room temperature (70° to 80°F.) until batter is above sides of pan, about 1½ hours. Preheat oven to 350°F.

5. Bake for 40 minutes, covering loosely with a sheet of aluminum foil after the first 25 minutes. Place on rack for 1 minute. Loosen around sides with blunt knife and carefully invert. Return inverted loaf to oven, and bake for 5 minutes (this ensures an all-over crispy crust). Place on rack to cool. Serve at room temperature, slightly warm, or toasted.

YIELD: About sixteen ⅜-inch slices

NOTE: An additional ¼ cup whole wheat flour may be substituted for ¼ cup buckwheat flour.

(55)K WHOLE-WHEAT POPOVERS

2 large eggs
1 cup skim milk
¾ cup sifted unbleached flour
¼ cup sifted whole-wheat pastry flour
1 tablespoon regular wheat germ

¼ teaspoon each salt and ground cinnamon
1 tablespoon oil
Sweet butter/margarine blend for baking cups

1. Preheat oven to 400°F. Place eggs and milk in blender. Blend on high speed for 5 seconds. Add remaining ingredients except shortening. Blend for 10 seconds. With rubber spatula, scrape down sides and bottom of blender. Blend until smooth, about 20 seconds.
2. Well grease six 5-ounce ovenproof custard cups. Place cups on jelly-roll pan. Half-fill each cup with batter. For well-baked brown crusted popovers, bake for 35 to 40 minutes. For light brown crusted popovers, reduce heat to 375°F. and bake for 45 to 50 minutes. Don't peek before prescribed time, or they'll all fall down.
3. Transfer cups to rack and let cool for 3 minutes. With blunt knife, carefully circle each cup around sides to loosen. Remove popovers.

YIELD: 6 large popovers

SERVING SUGGESTIONS: Serve with unsugared jam, or fill with scrambled eggs, or "bright" chicken, fish, meat, or vegetables.

VARIATIONS: Spiced Popovers: Add ¼ teaspoon each ground ginger and coriander (or cardamom) to batter in step 1.
Cheese Popovers: Sprinkle each batter-filled cup with 1 teaspoon freshly grated Parmesan or mozzarella cheese before baking.

NOTE: Two simple yet crucial things to remember when preparing popovers: The oven must be *preheated* to exact prescribed temperature, and the batter must be beaten to smooth perfection.

(56)K BACON-TASTING ONIONS AND EGGS

3 whole eggs
1 egg white
1 teaspoon smoked yeast (available in
 health-food stores)
⅛ teaspoon salt

2 tablespoons evaporated skim milk
¼ cup finely minced onions
1 tablespoon sweet butter/margarine
 blend
Freshly ground black pepper to taste

1. In small bowl, combine first 5 ingredients. Beat with fork to blend. Add onions. Beat again.
2. Heat butter/margarine blend in nonstick skillet over medium heat until bubbly. Add eggs. Cook for 2 to 3 seconds, then stir. Continue to stir while cooking until eggs are moist but hold their shape when stirring. Serve immediately, sprinkled with pepper to taste.

YIELD: Serves 2 to 3

(57) APPLE PANCAKE

1 teaspoon fresh lemon juice
2 medium Golden Delicious apples,
 peeled, cored, and thinly sliced
2 tablespoons date powder
½ teaspoon ground cinnamon
¼ teaspoon each ground ginger and
 freshly grated nutmeg or ground
 cardamom

4 tablespoons sweet butter/margarine
 blend
3 eggs, separated
2 tablespoons honey
½ cup evaporated skim milk
½ cup My Pancake Mix (page 174)

1. Pour lemon juice into bowl. Drop apples into bowl, turning to moisten. Sprinkle with date powder and spices; stir until evenly coated.
2. Melt 2 tablespoons shortening in 10-inch well-seasoned iron skillet, tilting skillet from side to side so that rim is moistened. Add apples, and over medium heat cook and stir until apples begin to soften, about 5 minutes. Remove skillet from heat.
3. In bowl, combine egg yolks, honey, and skim milk. Lightly beat with fork to blend. Stir in Pancake Mix.
4. Beat egg whites until stiff but not dry. Fold into pancake mixture (do not overfold). Preheat oven to 400°F.
5. Return skillet with apples to medium heat. Add remaining 2 tablespoons shortening and melt. Arrange apples in one layer. Spoon batter evenly over apples, taking care that edges are well covered. Place skillet in center section of oven and bake for 15 minutes.
6. Remove pancake from skillet by gently loosening edges with spatula, and inverting onto large plate. Cut into serving pieces, and serve immediately.

YIELD: Serves 4 to 5

(58) BLUEBERRY SAUCE

1 pint sweet fresh blueberries, rinsed
  and picked over (see Notes)
½ cup each unsweetened dark grape
  juice and apple juice
4 tablespoons My Fruit Butter (page
  178)

½ teaspoon ground cinnamon
1 2-inch piece vanilla bean, split
2 tablespoons honey

1. Place berries in 1½- to 2-quart heavy-bottomed saucepan. Partially crush with potato masher. Stir in balance of ingredients except honey. Bring to boil. Reduce heat and simmer, uncovered, for 15 minutes, stirring from time to time. Let cool. Stir in honey.
2. Remove vanilla bean, pressing out juices. Refrigerate in tightly closed glass jars. Serve chilled or at room temperature.

YIELD: 3 cups; serving size = ¼ cup

NOTES: Sweetness in berries will vary from box to box. If berries are particularly tart, increase honey to 3 tablespoons.

Sauce slightly thickens naturally after cooling. If thicker consistency is desired, dissolve 2 teaspoons arrowroot flour or cornstarch in 1 tablespoon cold water, and drizzle, while stirring, into hot mixture.

(59) JIFFY BLUEBERRY JAM

1½ cups Blueberry Sauce (see preceding
  recipe)
¼ cup unsweetened apple juice
2 tablespoons frozen orange or apple
  juice concentrate

1½ teaspoons unflavored gelatin
1 tablespoon honey

1. Cook Blueberry Sauce in heavy-bottomed saucepan over low heat to simmering point.
2. In cup, combine apple juice and frozen concentrate. Sprinkle with gelatin. Let stand for 3 minutes to soften. Add to hot sauce. Stir and simmer, uncovered, for 5 minutes. Let cool. Stir in honey.
3. Ladle into jars, cover tightly, and refrigerate for at least 2 hours. Mixture will thicken when chilled.

YIELD: About 1⅔ cups; serving size = 2 tablespoons

(60)K STUFFED PRUNES

1 tablespoon regular wheat germ
1 tablespoon finely chopped walnuts
½ teaspoon ground cinnamon

12 prunes (no preservatives added)
12 walnut halves
¼ cup unsweetened apple juice

1. In cup, combine wheat germ, chopped walnuts, and cinnamon, blending well. Sprinkle across sheet of waxed paper.
2. Slit each prune halfway through center and insert walnut halves. Squeeze to close.
3. Dip in apple juice, then roll in nut mixture. Chill.

YIELD: 12 prunes; serving size = up to 3 prunes

(61)K FROZEN YOGURT TUTTI-FRUITI

1 ripe banana
1 teaspoon fresh lemon juice
3 tablespoons unsalted smooth
    peanut butter
½ cup crushed unsweetened
    pineapple, drained

⅛ teaspoon ground cinnamon
2 dashes ground allspice
1½ cups low-fat plain yogurt
2 tablespoons honey

1. Place banana in bowl. Mash with fork. Sprinkle with lemon juice and mash again. Then blend in peanut butter, pineapple, and spices.
2. Fold in half of yogurt. Dribble in honey. Fold in remaining yogurt.
3. Pour into ice-cream maker, following manufacturer's directions, or pour into empty ice-cube trays. Turn refrigerator up to its coldest setting, cover tray, and freeze, stirring from time to time. After 1 hour, briskly whisk or beat with portable electric beater or rotary mixer. Return tray to freezer until mixture sets to desired consistency.

YIELD: About 1 pint; serving size = ½ cup

Bright Cuisine Dishes for Lunch

(62) BROCCOLI BISQUE

2 tablespoons corn oil
⅓ cup minced shallots or combination
    minced shallots and onions
4 cups fresh broccoli florets (1 large
    bunch)
1 tablespoon apple cider vinegar
2½ cups My "Canned" Chicken Broth
    (page 178) or broth made with
    low-sodium vegetable seasoning
½ cup unsweetened apple juice

1 tablespoon regular Cream of Wheat
1 tablespoon mild curry powder
½ teaspoon freshly grated nutmeg
¼ teaspoon salt
    Several sprigs parsley tied into
    bundle with white thread
3 tablespoons evaporated skim milk or
    regular skim milk
2 tablespoons grated carrot

1. Heat oil in heavy-bottomed 1½- to 2-quart saucepan until hot. Sauté shallots until wilted but not brown, stirring often. Add broccoli and sauté for 1 minute. Add vinegar and cook for 1 minute. Then add broth and apple juice. Bring to boil.
2. Sprinkle with Cream of Wheat. Stir in curry powder, half of nutmeg, and salt. Drop in parsley bundle. Reduce heat to simmering. Cover and simmer for 12 minutes, stirring once midway. Uncover and partially cool. Discard parsley bundle.
3. Pour mixture into blender, half at a time. Add remaining ¼ teaspoon nutmeg, and puree until smooth. Return to saucepan. Whisk in milk. Reheat to just under boiling point. Pour into serving dishes, sprinkle with carrot, and serve.

YIELD: Serves 5

(63) TOFU CASSEROLE—It's a Whole Meal!

1 pound eggplant, scrubbed, cut into
    ⅜-inch slices
2 tablespoons each corn and Italian
    olive oil, combined
2 tofu cakes (about ¾ pound)
1 cup chopped onions or combination
    of shallots and onion
2 tablespoons minced garlic
½ cup coarsely chopped sweet green
    pepper
¼ pound snow-white fresh
    mushrooms, trimmed, rinsed,
    dried, and thinly sliced

¼ teaspoon salt (optional)
½ teaspoon each dried marjoram and
    thyme leaves, crushed, and
    ground ginger
¼ cup My "Canned" Chicken Broth
    (page 178) or broth made with
    low-sodium vegetable seasoning
1½ cups crushed canned tomatoes
2 tablespoons unsweetened apple juice
¼ cup minced fresh parsley
¾ cup grated mozzarella cheese
    Freshly ground black pepper
    (optional)

1. Arrange eggplant slices on cookie sheet. Brush each side with 2 tablespoons oil. Broil under high heat until lightly browned on each side. Remove from broiler and set aside.
2. Cut tofu into ½-inch slices. Lay on double sheets of paper toweling. Blot with another sheet of toweling. Let drain.
3. Heat remaining 2 tablespoons oil over medium heat in nonstick skillet. Sauté onions (or onion and shallots), garlic, green pepper, and mushrooms until softened. In cup, combine salt, marjoram, thyme, and ginger. Sprinkle over mixture. Sauté for 1 minute. Add broth and cook for 1 minute. Then mix in tomatoes, apple juice, and parsley. Bring to simmering point. Simmer, uncovered, for 3 to 5 minutes, or until mixture is thick and most of liquid is reduced.
4. Preheat oven to 375°F. Assemble casserole in alternate layers of eggplant, tofu, tomato mixture, and cheese. Bake, uncovered, until lightly browned, 40 to 45 minutes. Sprinkle with freshly ground black pepper, if desired.

YIELD: Serves 4 to 5

(64)K VEAL BURGERS

1 pound lean ground veal
3 tablespoons finely minced shallot
2 tablespoons finely minced fresh
    parsley
1 teaspoon dried savory leaves,
    crushed
½ teaspoon chili con carne seasoning

1 teaspoon prepared Dijon mustard
1 tablespoon tomato paste
1 tablespoon reduced-sodium soy sauce
⅓ cup My Shake and Bake-Alike (page
    175)
1 tablespoon Italian olive oil

1. Place veal in bowl. Add 1 tablespoon shallot, 1 tablespoon parsley, savory leaves, and chili con carne seasoning. Blend well.
2. In cup, combine mustard with tomato paste and soy sauce. Add to meat and blend (your fingers will do the best job here). Shape into four ½-inch patties.
3. Sprinkle Shake and Bake-Alike across sheet of waxed paper. Press both sides of each patty into mixture.
4. Heat oil in well-seasoned iron skillet until hot. Spread remaining 2 tablespoons shallot across skillet. Sauté for 30 seconds over medium-high heat. Lay burgers atop shallots. Sauté on each side for 3 minutes. Burgers should be browned on the outside and lightly pink inside. Do not overcook. Serve immediately, sprinkle with remaining fresh parsley.

YIELD: Serves 4

(65) BARBECUED SWORDFISH

2 tablespoons fresh lemon juice
2 teaspoons wine vinegar
½ teaspoon dried thyme leaves, crushed
1 tablespoon Italian olive oil
1 tablespoon reduced-sodium soy sauce

1 tablespoon minced fresh parsley
1 teaspoon finely minced garlic
1 tablespoon finely minced shallot
1½ pounds swordfish, 1¼ inches thick, cut into serving pieces
Lemon wedges

1. Prepare marinade by combining in cup all ingredients except fish and lemon wedges and stirring to blend. Let stand for 10 minutes.
2. Place fish in shallow bowl. Pour marinade over both sides, pressing solids into fish. Cover and let marinate at room temperature for 1 to 2 hours. Prepare barbecue fire.
3. Place fish in meshed barbecue holder, so that it may be turned from one side to another without falling apart. Reserve any remaining marinade for basting.
4. If using charcoal, or mesquite, place barbecue holder on rack 4 to 5 inches from heat. If using an open-hearth broiler, set rack on high. Place barbecue holder on rack. Broil on each side for 5 minutes at a time, turning and spooning with reserved marinade every time fish is turned. Cooking time should be 20 to 30 minutes. Serve on warmed plates, and garnish with lemon wedges.

YIELD: Serves 4 to 5

NOTE: This marinade and cooking technique also works well with thick sliced halibut or salmon steaks.

(66) CHINESE-STYLE SAUTÉED SHRIMP

3 tablespoons cornstarch
½ teaspoon each ground ginger, dry mustard, and dried basil leaves, crushed
¼ teaspoon ground thyme
⅛ teaspoon each salt and cayenne pepper
1 teaspoon finely chopped lemon rind

1¼ pounds medium raw shrimp, shelled and deveined
1 tablespoon fresh lemon juice, plus juice from ½ lemon
2 tablespoons peanut oil
3 tablespoons finely minced shallot
½ teaspoon finely minced garlic
1 teaspoon reduced-sodium soy sauce

1. Prepare light coating first by combining cornstarch, seasonings, and lemon rind in bowl and blending well. Set aside.
2. Dry shrimp. Sprinkle with 1 tablespoon lemon juice, turning to evenly coat. Let stand at room temperature for 30 minutes.
3. Pat lightly with paper toweling. Add all of shrimp to bowl with coating and, using hands, toss and turn until shrimp are lightly coated.
4. Heat oil in large nonstick skillet. Spread shallot and garlic evenly across skillet. Sauté over medium-high heat for 1 minute. Lay shrimp atop mixture and sauté on each side until lightly browned, about 8 minutes total cooking time.
5. Sprinkle with soy sauce and juice of ½ lemon. Turn and sauté for 1 minute. Serve hot.

YIELD: Serves 4

(67)K VERSATILE SARDINE SALAD

1 4⅜-ounce can skinless and boneless sardines packed in water
1 tablespoon part-skim ricotta cheese
2 tablespoons fresh lemon juice
1½ teaspoons wine vinegar
2 to 3 tablespoons Italian olive oil
1½ teaspoons prepared Dijon mustard
½ teaspoon mild curry powder

½ teaspoon paprika, plus some for garnish
¼ cup finely chopped bean sprouts or celery
2 tablespoons minced shallot or onion
2 tablespoons finely minced fresh parsley
2 eggs, hard-cooked and mashed
Pinch salt

1. Drain sardines. Place in small bowl. Add cheese and mash.
2. In cup, combine lemon juice, vinegar, 2 tablespoons oil, mustard, and spices, beating with fork to blend. Stir into sardines. Then mix in balance of ingredients, using more oil if necessary to hold mixture together. Serve well chilled, sprinkled with paprika.

YIELD: Makes 16 hors d'oeuvres, 4 sandwiches, or 2 luncheon salads

(68) ROAST TURKEY THIGHS

2 turkey thighs, skinned (2½ to 2¾
    pounds)
¾ cup Cranberry-Spice Marinade (page
    248)

⅓ cup My "Canned" Chicken Broth
    (page 178) or broth made with
    low-sodium vegetable seasoning
2 tablespoons minced fresh parsley or
    coriander

1. Wash turkey. Dry thoroughly with paper toweling. Prick all over with sharp-pronged fork. Place in bowl. Spread with thick cranberry marinade. Cover and refrigerate for at least 4 hours or overnight, turning from time to time.
2. Preheat oven to 375°F. Lay thighs on rack in shallow roasting pan, reserving marinade that doesn't adhere. Cover tightly with aluminum foil. Roast for 20 minutes. Spoon with half of reserved marinade. Re-cover and roast for 40 minutes more. Turn. Re-cover and roast for 1¼ hours, or until fork-tender, turning and spooning with marinade once midway. (At end of cooking time, most of marinade will have evaporated.) Transfer to cutting board. Cover to keep warm.
3. Remove rack from roasting pan. Place pan over medium heat on top of stove. Add broth and parsley or coriander. Heat to boiling point, stirring to break up any crisp particles.
4. Slice turkey at an angle with sharp knife. Arrange on warmed individual plates, and spoon with small amount of hot sauce.

YIELD: Serves 4

SERVING SUGGESTION: Serve cold, thinly sliced, on whole-wheat bread.

(69) GINGER CHICKEN

4 teaspoons peeled and finely minced
    fresh ginger
1 tablespoon finely minced garlic
2 teaspoons corn or Italian olive oil
1 tablespoon fresh lime juice, plus
    juice of ½ lime
⅛ teaspoon each salt and black pepper

¼ teaspoon each mild curry powder and
    ground cumin
3 tablespoons thick buttermilk,
    preferably without salt added
1 3-pound broiling chicken, skinned,
    wing tips removed, cut into
    eighths
Minced fresh parsley

1. In cup, combine and blend ginger, garlic, oil, 1 tablespoon lime juice, and seasonings. Stir in buttermilk. Mixture will be thick.
2. Prick chicken all over with sharp-pronged fork. Place in bowl. Spread with ginger mixture, turning several times to coat. Cover and let marinate at room temperature for 1 hour.
3. Preheat oven to 375°F. Arrange chicken in one layer in shallow roasting pan. Cover loosely with aluminum foil. Roast for 30 minutes. Turn. Turn oven heat up to 400°F. Roast chicken, uncovered, for 20 minutes, turning and basting twice at equal intervals. Squeeze juice of ½ lime over chicken. Sprinkle with parsley and serve.

YIELD: Serves 4 to 5

SERVING SUGGESTION: Serve cold, thinly sliced, on whole-wheat bread.

(70) PASTA AND BEANS

2 cups cooked pinto beans
2 cups just-cooked elbow
   macaroni or small pasta
   shells, cooked al dente
½ teaspoon each ground cumin
   and mild curry powder
¼ teaspoon salt
2 tablespoons Italian olive oil
¾ cup coarsely chopped scallions
1 large sweet red pepper, seeded
   and julienned
1 tablespoon minced garlic

2 tablespoons balsamic vinegar
⅔ cup My "Canned" Chicken
   Broth (page 178) or broth
   made with low-sodium
   vegetable seasoning
½ to ¾ cup tomato puree (no salt
   added)
2 tablespoons each minced fresh
   parsley and dill
   Freshly ground black pepper to
   taste
   Freshly grated Parmesan cheese

1. In large bowl, place beans and pasta. Sprinkle and gently toss with spices and salt.
2. Heat oil in large nonstick skillet until hot. Over medium heat, sauté scallions, red pepper, and garlic until wilted. Add bean mixture. Sauté while stirring until heated through. Pour vinegar around sides of skillet. Cook and stir for 1 minute.
3. Combine broth with ½ cup tomato puree. Pour around sides of skillet. When bubbling, stir into solids. Cover and simmer for 5 minutes, adding remaining tomato puree to taste, if desired.
4. Stir in fresh parsley and dill. Turn into serving bowl. Sprinkle with freshly ground pepper and Parmesan cheese.

YIELD: 5 to 6 main course servings

VARIATION: Stir in ½ cup cooked diced chicken or meat in step 3.

(71)K BROCCOLI-CHICKEN SALAD

1 cup cooked chopped broccoli
1 cup cooked chicken, cut into ½-inch
   pieces
1 medium onion, finely chopped
¼ cup tomato puree
2 teaspoons fresh lemon juice

2 tablespoons Light Mayonnaise (page
   182)
¼ cup finely grated Parmesan cheese
⅛ teaspoon freshly grated nutmeg
2 tablespoons minced fresh parsley or
   dill or a combination of both

1. Place broccoli and chicken in bowl. Add onion and toss.
2. In cup, combine and blend tomato puree, lemon juice, and mayonnaise.
   Fold into chicken mixture. Sprinkle with Parmesan and nutmeg, and gently
   stir.
3. Serve as sandwich filling or as salad, sprinkled with parsley or dill.

YIELD: About 2¼ cups

(72)K COLORFUL SALAD WITH FRUIT DRESSING

Salad:

8 lettuce cups
1 cup loosely packed alfalfa sprouts

¾ cup coarsely grated unpeeled
   zucchini
¾ cup finely grated carrot

Fruit Dressing:

½ teaspoon prepared Dijon mustard
3 tablespoons frozen orange juice
   concentrate
1½ teaspoons My Spicy Mix (page
   177)

⅓ cup apple cider vinegar
2 tablespoons oil
½ teaspoon honey

1. Arrange lettuce cups on 4 salad plates. Fill, in layers, with equal amounts
   of sprouts and zucchini, topping with carrots.
2. In small bowl, whisk first 4 dressing ingredients until well blended. Then
   whisk in oil and honey. Serve in sauceboat with salad.

YIELD: Serves 4; Fruit Dressing alone: ⅔ cup (serving size = up to 3 tablespoons)

(73) SAUTÉED APPLES AND ZUCCHINI

1 tablespoon corn oil
1 small onion, halved, thinly sliced,
  and separated into rings
3 medium zucchini (about 1 pound),
  ends trimmed, well scrubbed, and
  cut into ⅜-inch slices
2 Golden Delicious apples, cored,
  peeled, halved, and cut into ⅜-
  inch slices

1 teaspoon My Spicy Mix (page 177)
¼ teaspoon salt
1 teaspoon apple cider vinegar
⅓ cup low-fat plain yogurt
2 tablespoons minced fresh basil or dill

1. Heat oil in large nonstick skillet until hot. Add onion and sauté over medium heat for 2 minutes. Add zucchini and apples. Sauté for 2 minutes,
   stirring continually. Sprinkle with Spicy Mix and salt.
2. Sauté until crisp-tender over medium-high heat, about 3 minutes. Add vinegar and quickly stir. Remove from heat.
3. Stir in yogurt. Place skillet over low heat and cook until just under simmering point. Turn into serving dish. Sprinkle with basil or dill, and serve hot,
   or chill and serve as relish or salad.

YIELD: Serves 4 to 5

(74)K   PEANUT BUTTER MILK SHAKE

3 ice cubes, crushed
½ cup skim milk
¼ cup unsweetened pineapple juice
1 tablespoon unsalted peanut butter

1 ripe peach or small banana, or ½ cup
  fresh berries in season
1 teaspoon honey (optional)

Place all ingredients in blender. Blend on high speed for 1 minute. Serve at
once.

YIELD: Serves 1

VARIATION: The addition of a pinch of ground ginger, cinnamon, or cardamom
or any combination is a flavor booster (for fruit milk shakes, too).

(75) APPLESAUCE PUDDING SQUARES

1¾ cups My Muffin and Cake Mix
(page 172)
½ teaspoon each ground ginger and
cinnamon
⅛ teaspoon ground allspice
¼ teaspoon freshly grated nutmeg
2 tablespoons each corn oil and sweet
butter/margarine blend
4 tablespoons My Fruit Butter (page
178)

1 tablespoon honey
1 egg
1¾ cups Applesauce (page 203)
¼ cup low-fat plain yogurt
⅓ cup dark raisins
¼ cup coarsely chopped almonds or
walnuts
¾ teaspoon pure vanilla extract

1. Combine Muffin and Cake Mix with spices. Set aside.
2. Combine oil, shortening, Fruit Butter, and honey in large bowl of mixing machine. Beat until blended. Add egg and beat for 1 minute on medium speed.
3. Combine applesauce and yogurt and add to mixture alternately with dry ingredients. Stir in raisins, nuts, and vanilla.
4. Preheat oven to 350°F. and grease a 9-inch square pan. Bake for 65 minutes. Top should be golden brown and toothpick inserted in center should come out clean.
5. Place pan on rack and cool for 15 minutes. Cut into 16 squares. Serve warm.

YIELD: 16 squares

(76)K APPLE SAUTÉ

2 tablespoons sweet butter/margarine
blend
4 crisp sweet apples, such as
Washington State or Golden
Delicious, cored, peeled, and
thinly sliced
¼ teaspoon each ground cardamom and
ginger

½ teaspoon ground cinnamon
2 tablespoons chopped blanched
almonds or pine nuts
2 tablespoons date powder
2 teaspoons fresh lemon juice
2 tablespoons unsweetened apple juice
1 teaspoon unsulphured blackstrap
molasses or honey

1. Over medium-high heat, melt 1 tablespoon shortening in nonstick skillet. Add apples. Sauté and stir for 2 minutes.
2. Sprinkle with spices, nuts, and date powder. Stir and sauté for 2 minutes. Add remaining shortening, turning apples to coat. Sauté for 2 more minutes.

3. Combine lemon juice with apple juice and molasses or honey. Pour around sides of skillet. Cook and stir until apples are lightly browned and crisp-tender. Serve at once.

Yield: Serves 4

Serving suggestions: Top with low-fat plain yogurt, Dessert Topping (page 224), Choc-O-Chip Ice Milk (page 260), or Beige Ice Cream (recipe follows).

(77) BEIGE ICE CREAM

1 cup skim milk
¾ cup evaporated skim milk
1 1-inch piece vanilla bean, split
¼ teaspoon ground cinnamon
Dash ground allspice

2 tablespoons grain coffee
Dash salt
2 egg yolks
2 tablespoons honey

1. Bring some water in bottom of double boiler to boil. Reduce heat to simmering. In top of double boiler combine and stir all ingredients except egg yolks and honey. Cook for 5 minutes, stirring often.
2. In cup, lightly beat egg yolks with fork. Pour about ¼ cup hot liquid into cup and blend. Pour mixture back into pot and cook until it coats back of spoon, about 4 minutes. Remove from heat. Press out juices from vanilla bean, and discard bean. Let cool, whisking occasionally. Stir in honey.
3. Pour into ice-cream maker, following manufacturer's directions, or pour into empty ice-cube trays. Turn refrigerator up to its coldest setting. Cover tray and freeze, stirring from time to time. After 1 hour, briskly whisk or beat with portable electric beater or rotary mixer. Return tray to freezer until ice cream sets to desired consistency.

Yield: About 1 pint; serving size = ½ cup

Bright Cuisine Dishes for Dinner

(78) NEW-FASHIONED MUSHROOM AND BARLEY SOUP

½ ounce imported dried mushrooms,
 preferably dark variety
1¼ cups water
½ pound lean beef, such as top round,
 cut into ¼-inch pieces
3 teaspoons My Spicy Mix (page
 177)
2 tablespoons Italian olive or corn oil
1½ cups My Frozen Vegetable Mix
 (page 173)

4 teaspoons balsamic vinegar
3 cups My "Canned" Chicken Broth
 (page 178) or broth made with
 low-sodium vegetable seasoning
1 teaspoon low-sodium vegetable
 seasoning
2 tablespoons tomato paste
¼ cup barley, rinsed

1. Rinse mushrooms under running water. Break into small pieces. Place in cup. Add ¼ cup water, and soak for 30 minutes.
2. Sprinkle meat with 1½ teaspoons Spicy Mix, working well with hands into meat. Heat oil until hot in 1½- to 2-quart heavy-bottomed saucepan. Add meat, and quickly sear, stirring and cooking for 1 minute. Reduce heat to moderate. Add Vegetable Mix. Stir and cook until vegetables begin to soften, about 3 minutes.
3. Stir in vinegar. Cook for 1 minute. Add balance of water and remaining ingredients, and mushrooms with soaking liquid. Bring to boil. Reduce heat to simmering. Cover and cook for 1½ hours, stirring from time to time. Remove from heat and let stand for 10 minutes, covered, before serving.

YIELD: Serves 5

(79) THREE MARINADES

The quickest and simplest way to season chicken, Cornish hen, and bland cuts of meat is with marinades. Preparation time never exceeds 5 minutes, and the dish soaks up flavors unattended until you're ready to pop it into your oven or onto your broiler or outdoor grill.

(79A) BARBECUE MARINADE

1 tablespoon frozen apple juice
 concentrate
2 tablespoons oil
1 tablespoon honey
2 teaspoons tomato paste
1 tablespoon balsamic or wine vinegar

2 teaspoons My Spicy Mix (page 177)
1 tablespoon minced dried onions
¼ cup My "Canned" Chicken Broth
 (page 178) or broth made with
 low-sodium vegetable seasoning

1. Place frozen concentrate and oil in bowl. Blend, crushing concentrate with spoon until softened. Add honey, tomato paste, and vinegar, blending well.
2. Stir in remaining ingredients. Cover and let stand at room temperature for 15 minutes before using.

YIELD: About ¾ cup—enough to marinate a 3-pound chicken, roast, or 2½ to 3 pounds turkey parts.

(79B) INDIAN-STYLE MARINADE

¼ cup chopped shallots or onion
2 teaspoons minced garlic
1 tablespoon each apple cider vinegar and balsamic vinegar
1 tablespoon oil
1½ teaspoons dried rosemary leaves, crushed

½ teaspoon each mild curry powder, ground ginger, and cumin
¼ teaspoon salt
¼ cup plain yogurt

1. Combine all ingredients, except yogurt, in bowl. Stir to blend. Let stand for 5 minutes.
2. Gently stir in yogurt. Mixture will be thick. Cover and let stand at room temperature for 10 minutes before using.

YIELD: About ¾ cup—enough to marinate a 3-pound chicken, roast, or 2½ to 3 pound of turkey parts

(79C) CRANBERRY-SPICE MARINADE

2 tablespoons frozen orange juice concentrate
2 tablespoons corn or Italian olive oil
¼ cup wine vinegar
1 tablespoon each peeled and finely minced fresh ginger and garlic
2 tablespoons finely minced shallot

½ teaspoon each ground cumin, mild curry powder, dried sage leaves, and chili con carne seasoning
¼ teaspoon salt
½ cup fresh cranberries, well rinsed, picked over, and chopped (see Note)

1. Place frozen concentrate and oil in bowl. Blend, crushing concentrate with spoon until softened.
2. Stir in remaining ingredients. Mixture will be thick. Cover and let stand at room temperature for 15 minutes before using.

YIELD: About ¾ cup—enough to marinate a 3-pound chicken, roast, or 2½ to 3 pounds of turkey parts

NOTE: Rolling cranberries can be quickly chopped in electric mini-chopper or food processor.

(80) CHICKEN WITH APPLES

2 tablespoons oil
1 cup My Frozen Vegetable Mix (page 173)
⅛ pound fresh mushrooms, ends trimmed, rinsed, dried, and coarsely chopped
1 3-pound broiling chicken, skinned, wing tips removed, cut into eighths
2 tablespoons My Spicy Mix (page 177)

1 tablespoon apple cider vinegar
1 tablespoon tomato paste
1 tablespoon reduced-sodium soy sauce
½ cup each tomato juice, preferably low-sodium, and apple juice
⅛ teaspoon salt
2 Golden Delicious apples, cored, peeled, and sliced

1. Heat oil in well-seasoned iron skillet or Dutch oven until hot. Add Vegetable Mix and mushrooms. Cook, stirring, until softened, about 5 minutes. Spread mixture across skillet.
2. Sprinkle and rub chicken with Spicy Mix. Lay atop sautéed mixture in one layer. Cook for 5 minutes over medium-high heat without turning. Turn. Cook for 5 minutes more.
3. Pour vinegar around sides of skillet. Cook for 1 minute.
4. In cup, combine and blend tomato paste, soy sauce, tomato juice, and apple juice. Pour around sides of skillet. Sprinkle with salt (omit if regular tomato juice is used). Bring to boil. Spoon sauce and turn chicken parts to coat. Reduce heat to simmering. Cover and simmer for 65 minutes, turning twice and spooning with sauce at equal intervals.
5. Add apples, pushing into sauce. Re-cover and cook for 15 minutes.
6. With slotted spoon, transfer chicken to large serving plate. Cover to keep warm. Place skillet over medium-high heat. Reduce sauce, stirring until thickened, about 4 minutes. Spoon sauce and apples over chicken and serve at once.

YIELD: Serves 4

(81) POACHED CHICKEN WITH CREAMY SAUCE

Chicken:

2 small boned and skinned
chicken breasts (about 1¼
pounds), each breast
halved
1 small rib celery, coarsely
chopped
1 small onion, coarsely
chopped
2 tablespoons grated carrot

2 sprigs parsley and 1 bay leaf
wrapped into neat bundle
and tied with white thread
About 1½ cups My "Canned" Chicken
Broth (page 178) or broth
made with low-sodium
vegetable seasoning
Watercresss sprigs for
garnish

Creamy Sauce:

2 teaspoons sweet butter/
margarine blend
1 tablespoon finely minced
shallot
4 teaspoons unbleached flour
½ to ¾ cup poaching liquid
½ teaspoon each dried sage
leaves and mild curry
powder

3 tablespoons evaporated skim
milk
2 tablespoons freshly grated
Parmesan cheese
1 tablespoon minced fresh
parsley
⅛ teaspoon salt
Cayenne pepper to taste
¼ to ½ teaspoon fresh lemon juice

1. Wash and dry chicken thoroughly. Place in wide pan or nonstick skillet large enough to hold serving pieces in one layer. Strew with vegetables. Drop in parsley bundle. Add enough broth to barely cover. Bring to boil. Reduce heat to simmering. Cover and simmer for 20 minutes, spooning with broth twice at equal intervals.
2. With slotted spoon, transfer chicken to hot platter. Cover to keep warm. Strain ¾ cup poaching broth into measuring cup, reserving remaining broth for another dish.
3. Over medium heat, cook butter/margarine blend in heavy-bottomed small saucepan (preferably enameled) until melted. Add shallot and sauté without browning for 1 minute. Stir in flour with wooden spoon and cook over low heat for 1 minute. Whisk in ½ cup poaching broth. Cook until thickened. Sprinkle in sage and curry powder. Whisk and cook over low heat for 1 minute.
4. Add milk, cheese, and parsley. Cook and stir with whisk for 2 minutes. Pour any juices that have drained from chicken into sauce. Use remaining ¼ cup broth to thin down sauce to desired consistency.
5. Sprinkle with salt, cayenne pepper, and ¼ teaspoon lemon juice, whisking to blend. Cook for 30 seconds. Taste. Add more cayenne and/or lemon

juice, if desired. Pour over chicken. Garnish with watercress, and serve at once.

YIELD: Serves 4; Creamy Sauce: 1 scant cup

(82) ROAST CHICKEN WITH ROSY SAUCE

4 chicken legs with thighs (about 2½ pounds), skinned and disjointed
3 tablespoons finely minced shallot
1 tablespoon each peeled and finely minced fresh ginger and garlic
2 tablespoons balsamic vinegar
1 tablespoon wine vinegar
1 tablespoon frozen orange or pineapple juice concentrate
1 tablespoon My Spicy Mix (page 177)
1 tablespoon Italian olive oil

6 tablespoons My "Canned" Chicken Broth (page 178) or broth made with low-sodium vegetable seasoning
3 large snow-white fresh mushrooms, ends trimmed, rinsed, dried, and thinly sliced
1 tablespoon arrowroot flour dissolved in 1 tablespoon water
1 tablespoon minced fresh parsley
Black pepper to taste

1. Prick chicken with sharp-pronged fork. Place in bowl.
2. Prepare marinade by combining in cup shallot, ginger, garlic, vinegars, juice, Spicy Mix, oil, and 2 tablespoons broth, stirring well to blend. Pour over chicken, turning many times to coat. Cover and let marinate for at least 1 hour at room temperature, spooning with marinade several times.
3. Preheat oven to 375°F. Transfer chicken to shallow roasting pan, spooning with marinade. Cover loosely with sheet of aluminum foil. Roast for 20 minutes. Uncover and turn. Spoon with marinade. Return to oven, uncovered, for 30 to 40 minutes, turning and spooning with marinade once midway. Transfer to warmed serving plate. Cover to keep warm.
4. Pour marinade into measuring cup. There should be about ⅔ cup. If not, add additional broth to bring measurement up to ⅔ cup. Pour into heavy-bottomed saucepan. Add remaining ¼ cup broth and mushrooms. Bring to boil. Reduce heat, partially cover, and simmer for 5 minutes. Dribble in arrowroot mixture, using only enough to lightly thicken sauce. Sprinkle with parsley, and simmer for 1 minute while stirring. Add pepper to taste. Spoon over chicken and serve at once.

YIELD: Serves 4 to 5

(83) STEWED CHICKEN WITH APRICOTS

4 chicken legs with thighs (about 2½
   pounds), skinned and disjointed
2 teaspoons My Spicy Mix (page 177)
⅛ teaspoon salt
2 tablespoons cornstarch
5 teaspoons Italian olive oil
1 tablespoon finely minced garlic
1 medium sweet green pepper, seeded
   and julienned

¼ pound snow-white fresh mushrooms,
   ends trimmed, rinsed, dried, and
   coarsely chopped
1 tablespoon apple cider vinegar
⅔ cup canned crushed tomatoes
¼ cup unsweetened apple juice
1 thin lemon slice
½ cup well-rinsed coarsely chopped
   dried apricots (without
   preservatives added)

1. Rinse chicken and dry thoroughly with paper toweling. Prick all over with sharp-pronged fork.
2. In cup, combine and blend Spicy Mix, salt, and cornstarch. Spread over sheet of waxed paper. Roll chicken in mixture, pressing to adhere.
3. Heat 3 teaspoons oil in well-seasoned iron skillet until hot. Using medium-high heat, brown chicken on both sides. Transfer to plate.
4. Spread remaining 2 teaspoons oil over skillet. Add garlic, green pepper, and mushrooms. Stir and sauté until wilted, adjusting heat so that mixture doesn't brown.
5. Add vinegar. Cook for 30 seconds. Add balance of ingredients. Bring to simmering point and cook for 1 minute. Return browned chicken to skillet, turning several times to coat. Cover and simmer for 45 to 50 minutes, or until fork-tender, turning and spooning with sauce 4 times at equal intervals.
6. Remove skillet from heat and let stand, covered, for 10 minutes before serving. Sauce will be thick and chicken will have an all-over glossy appearance.

YIELD: Serves 4

(84) SCALLOP OF VEAL

2 *tablespoons each unbleached flour*
   and fine toasted bread crumbs,
   preferably homemade (page 217)
2 *tablespoons freshly grated Parmesan*
   cheese
¼ *teaspoon each salt and ground thyme*
½ *teaspoon dry mustard*
1 *teaspoon each dried basil and*
   oregano leaves, crushed
1 *pound veal scaloppine, cut from the*
   leg, flattened to ⅛-inch thickness

2 *tablespoons plus 1 teaspoon Italian*
   olive oil
3 *tablespoons minced shallot*
½ *cup minced snow-white fresh*
   mushrooms
2 *teaspoons balsamic vinegar*
¾ *cup My "Canned" Chicken Broth*
   (page 178) or broth made with
   low-sodium vegetable seasoning
½ *lemon*
   Minced fresh parsley or basil

1. Prepare coating mix by combining and blending flour, bread crumbs, cheese, and seasonings in bowl. Spread half of mixture across sheet of waxed paper.
2. Rinse and dry veal well. Lay atop flour mixture, pressing to adhere. Spoon remaining coating over meat, pressing to adhere.
3. Prepare veal in 2 batches. Heat 1 tablespoon oil in well-seasoned iron skillet until hot. Over medium-high heat, sauté half the veal on each side for about 2 minutes, or until lightly browned. Transfer to plate. Add 1 tablespoon oil to skillet. Brown remaining veal. Transfer to plate.
4. Spread remaining 1 teaspoon oil across skillet. Add shallot and mushrooms. Sauté, scraping pan with spatula to loosen crisp particles. Cook until wilted.
5. Pour vinegar around sides of skillet. Stir to combine. Cook for 1 minute. Add broth and bring to boil. Reduce heat and simmer for 2 minutes.
6. Return veal to skillet. Spoon several times with sauce. Cook until just heated through. Sprinkle with lemon juice. Arrange on warmed serving plates, sprinkled with minced parsley or basil.

YIELD: Serves 4 to 5

VARIATION: If you have My Shake and Bake-Alike (page 175) on your shelf, substitute ½ cup for all the coating ingredients.

(85) **BRAISED VEAL**

1 *teaspoon dried sage leaves*	1 *tablespoon wine vinegar*
½ *teaspoon ground thyme*	½ *cup My "Canned" Chicken Broth*
⅛ *teaspoon salt*	*(page 178) or broth made with*
3 *pounds boneless veal roast, rolled*	*low-sodium vegetable seasoning*
and tied to 5-inch diameter	1½ *cups crushed tomatoes*
2 *tablespoons Italian olive oil*	1½ *teaspoons reduced-sodium soy sauce*
1½ *cups My Frozen Vegetable Mix*	1 *tablespoon frozen orange juice*
(page 173)	*concentrate*

1. In cup, combine sage, thyme, and salt. Prick meat all over with sharp-pronged fork or with tip of sharp knife. Sprinkle and rub with seasoning.
2. Heat oil in heavy casserole until hot. Lightly brown meat, rolling to brown evenly. Transfer to plate.
3. Add Vegetable Mix to casserole. Stir and cook for 3 minutes. Add vinegar. Cook for 30 seconds. Add balance of ingredients. Bring to simmering point and simmer for 2 minutes. Return meat to pot, turning several times to coat. Spoon with sauce. Cover and simmer over very low heat for 2 to 2½ hours, or until fork-tender, rolling meat and spooning with sauce from time to time.
4. Transfer meat to carving board. Remove strings. Tent with aluminum foil and let stand for 8 to 10 minutes. Cut with very sharp knife, and arrange on warm serving plate. Skim any fat from sauce and reheat. Spoon small amount of sauce over each slice of meat. Serve remaining sauce in sauceboat.

YIELD: Serves 6 to 8

NOTE: Flavor is improved and meat can be thinly cut when dish is prepared a day ahead. Store cooked meat and sauce in separate tightly closed containers. When ready to reheat, remove strings from meat, thinly slice, and place slices in nonstick skillet. Cut away any congealed fat from top of sauce. Add one-third of sauce to skillet. Cook over low heat until heated through. Heat remaining sauce in saucepan. Serve veal on individual warm plates with extra sauce in sauceboat.

(86) LAMB PATTIES

1 pound lamb, cut from the shank,
    well trimmed, cut into chunks
1 tablespoon My Spicy Mix (page
    177)
2 tablespoons balsamic or wine vinegar
¼ cup My Shake and Bake-Alike (page
    175) or fine-toasted homemade
    bread crumbs (page 217)

1 tablespoon tomato paste
4 average size shallots, peeled and
    halved
¼ cup tightly packed parsley florets
1 tablespoon finely grated Parmesan
    cheese
⅛ teaspoon salt
1 tablespoon Italian olive oil

1. Fit food processor with steel blade. Place all ingredients in processor. Process until mixture is well chopped. Shape into 4 patties. Cover and refrigerate for 1 hour.
2. Heat oil in nonstick skillet until hot. Sauté burgers on each side until browned and slightly pink inside, 7 to 8 minutes. Serve immediately.

YIELD: Serves 4

NOTE: For alternate cooking methods (broiling and barbecue), see the recipe for Whamburger (page 191).

(87) MIXED MEAT STEW

1 pound each lean beef round and lean
    pork fillets, cut into 1-inch cubes
1 tablespoon My Spicy Mix (page
    177)
2 tablespoons Italian olive oil
2 cups My Frozen Vegetable Mix
    (page 173)
1 tablespoon balsamic vinegar

1 cup crushed tomatoes
⅛ teaspoon salt
1 thin slice lemon
2 bay leaves, wrapped in washed
    cotton cheesecloth and tied with
    white thread
Minced fresh parsley or dill or a
    combination of both

1. Wipe meat with paper toweling. Sprinkle with Spicy Mix, working in with hands.
2. Heat oil in heavy casserole until hot. Add Vegetable Mix. Over medium-high heat, stir and cook for 3 minutes. Add meat, combine with Vegetable Mix, and cook, stirring, until meat loses its pink color, about 5 minutes.
3. Add vinegar. Cook for 1 minute. Stir in tomatoes, salt, and lemon slice; drop in bay leaf bundle. Bring to simmering point. Reduce heat. Cover and simmer until fork-tender, about 1½ hours, stirring from time to time. Discard bay leaf bundle and lemon slice. Stir. Re-cover and let stand for 30 minutes before serving, reheating briefly if necessary.
4. Ladle into serving bowl, and sprinkle with parsley or dill or a combination of both.

YIELD: Serves 5 to 6

SERVING SUGGESTION: Delicious served over a bed of just-cooked brown rice or orzo pasta.

(88) SHRIMP WITH BANANA

3 tablespoons cornstarch
½ teaspoon ground ginger
¼ teaspoon each ground cinnamon and coriander
3 dashes cayenne pepper
¼ teaspoon salt
1 pound shrimp, shelled, deveined, and well dried
6 teaspoons peanut oil

3 tablespoons each minced shallot and sweet green pepper
1 large almost-ripe banana, cut into ½-inch dice
3 tablespoons apple cider vinegar
¼ cup My "Canned" Chicken Broth (page 178) or broth made with low-sodium vegetable seasoning
½ cup unsweetened pineapple juice
1 tablespoon fresh lemon juice

1. In bowl, combine cornstarch with spices and salt. Add shrimp, turning to coat. Set aside.
2. Heat 4½ teaspoons oil in well-seasoned iron skillet. Sauté shallot and green pepper until wilted but not brown, about 2 minutes. Arrange shrimp atop sautéed ingredients. Sauté for 1½ minutes on each side. Push all ingredients to side of skillet.
3. Add remaining 1½ teaspoons oil to skillet. Sauté banana, stirring continually for 1 minute. Then gently combine with shrimp mixture. Sprinkle with vinegar. Stir and cook for 30 seconds.
4. Combine broth with pineapple juice. Pour around side of skillet. Simmer until sauce thickens, about 1½ minutes, spooning shrimp with sauce.
5. Sprinkle with lemon juice and stir. Serve at once over a bed of just-cooked rice.

YIELD: Serves 4

(89) FILLET OF SOLE IN FRUIT SAUCE

1 tablespoon fresh lemon juice
1 teaspoon frozen orange juice concentrate
½ teaspoon My Spicy Mix (page 177)
3 tablespoons milk
1¼ pounds fillet of sole, cut into serving pieces (see Note)
2 tablespoons minced shallot

1 tablespoon sweet butter/margarine blend, cut into small pieces
2 tablespoons freshly grated Parmesan cheese
1 tablespoon fine toasted bread crumbs (page 217)
Minced fresh parsley
Lemon wedges

1. In bowl, combine first 4 ingredients, beating with fork to blend.
2. Wash and dry fish thoroughly. Add to liquid mixture, turning several times to coat. Let marinate for at least 30 minutes at room temperature, or cover and refrigerate for several hours.
3. Arrange fish in broiling pan in one layer. Pour marinade over it. Sprinkle with shallot. Then dot with butter/margarine blend. Broil fairly close to heat for 8 minutes. Spoon with sauce. Sprinkle with cheese, crumbs, and parsley. Return to broiler for about 4 minutes, or until fish is lightly browned. Serve immediately, garnished with lemon wedges.

YIELD: Serves 4

NOTES: You can use fillets of lemon sole, gray sole, flounder, or sea bass.

A French chef's recipe for fish usually reads: "Cook until just springy to the touch." Many Americans, my husband and I included, like their fish cooked longer. If you and your family are among this group, cook fish until it flakes easily when tested with a fork.

(90) NEW COLESLAW

1 ½-pound wedge cabbage, steamed for 3 minutes, cooled
1 small onion
½ medium sweet green or red pepper, seeded
2 ribs celery
1 8-ounce can sliced beets, preferably without salt added
1 Golden Delicious apple, cored, peeled, and quartered
⅓ cup tightly packed flat fresh parsley or just-snipped dill

2 tablespoons each apple cider vinegar and fresh lemon juice
1 teaspoon low-sodium vegetable seasoning or My Seasoning Mix (page 176)
¼ teaspoon salt
¼ cup buttermilk, preferably without salt added
3 tablespoons Light Mayonnaise (page 182)

1. Use food processor fitted with steel blade. Cut cooled cabbage into chunks. Place in workbowl and process on/off twice.
2. Cut onion, pepper, and celery into uniform pieces and add to workbowl. Process on/off once.
3. Add beets, apple, and parsley or dill. Process on/off 3 or 4 times, or until mixture is chopped. Turn into large bowl.
4. Sprinkle and stir in vinegar, lemon juice, vegetable seasoning or Seasoning Mix, and salt.
5. Stir in buttermilk. Then gently fold in mayonnaise, a tablespoon at a time. Cover bowl and chill for at least 2 hours before serving, gently stirring twice at equal intervals.

YIELD: 1 quart; serving size = up to ¾ cup

(91) CORN AND PEPPERS

3 fresh ears of small-kerneled corn,
  cleaned
1 tablespoon oil
1 small sweet red pepper, seeded and
  julienned
2 tablespoons minced shallot
½ teaspoon ground ginger

¼ teaspoon ground marjoram
⅛ teaspoon salt
1 teaspoon apple cider vinegar
2 tablespoons minced fresh basil, dill,
  or parsley
Black pepper, freshly ground
  preferred (optional)

1. Steam corn until tender, about 10 minutes. Stand cobs upright on cutting board. With serrated knife, cut kernels from cob.
2. Heat oil in nonstick skillet until hot. Sauté sweet red pepper and shallot until just wilted (do not brown). Add corn, stirring to combine.
3. Sprinkle with ginger, marjoram, and salt. Stir and sauté for 30 seconds. Add vinegar and cook until all ingredients are heated through. Stir in fresh basil, dill, or parsley. Sprinkle with pepper, if desired, and serve at once.

YIELD: Serves 4

(92) FAST AND SIMPLE KASHA (BUCKWHEAT GROATS)

2 cups My "Canned" Chicken Broth
  (page 178) or broth made with
  low-sodium vegetable seasoning
2 teaspoons My Spicy Mix (page 177)
3 large snow-white fresh mushrooms,
  ends trimmed, rinsed, dried, and
  coarsely chopped

2 tablespoons finely minced carrot
1 cup whole kasha
¼ cup coarsely chopped scallions
1 tablespoon sweet butter/margarine
  blend
1 tablespoon minced fresh parsley or
  dill

1. In 1½- to 2-quart heavy-bottomed saucepan, combine Chicken Broth, Spicy Mix, mushrooms, and carrot. Bring to rolling boil.
2. Add kasha and stir. Bring to boil again. Reduce heat to medium boil. Cook, uncovered, for exactly 8 minutes, stirring often, particularly at end of prescribed cooking time. All liquid will be absorbed. Remove from heat.
3. Stir in scallions and butter/margarine blend. Cover and let stand for 5 minutes. Fluff up with fork and serve, sprinkled with parsley, dill, or any fresh minced herb of your choice.

YIELD: 3 cups; serves 4 to 6

VARIATION: After stirring in scallions and shortening (step 3), add ½ cup crushed tomatoes. Simmer, uncovered, for 3 minutes. Sprinkle with 2 tablespoons freshly grated Parmesan cheese, then sprinkle with minced fresh herb of your choice.

(93) POTATO PANCAKES

1 *large egg*
2 *tablespoons skim milk*
⅛ *teaspoon each salt, black pepper, and ground cinnamon*
¼ *cup finely grated carrot*

2 *tablespoons grated onion*
1 *pound baking potatoes*
½ *cup My Pancake Mix (page 174)*
6 *teaspoons oil*

1. In bowl, combine egg, milk, salt, pepper, and cinnamon, beating with fork to blend. Stir in carrot and onion.
2. Grate potatoes, draining off any liquid. Add to bowl. Sprinkle with Pancake Mix. Stir only until blended.
3. Spread 2 teaspoons oil across well-seasoned iron skillet. Place over medium-high heat until drip of cold water dropped into skillet bounces off. Arrange 4 pancakes in each batch using a heaping tablespoon of batter for each pancake. Flatten each pancake to 4 inches. Cook until brown on both sides, about 6 minutes, adjusting heat if necessary to maintain constant heat.
4. Transfer to warm plate and serve one lucky person immediately, or keep pancakes warm, uncovered, in 300°F. oven, while remaining 2 batches are prepared.

YIELD: 12 pancakes; serving size = 2 to 3 pancakes

(94) EGGPLANT "CAVIAR"

1 *pound eggplant, well scrubbed*
¾ *pound ripe tomatoes*
1 *tablespoon minced garlic*
½ *cup minced onion or shallot*
2 *tablespoons minced fresh dill or parsley*
2 *tablespoons fresh lemon juice*

1 *tablespoon red wine vinegar*
2 *teaspoons tomato paste*
½ *teaspoon mild curry powder*
⅛ *teaspoon each cayenne pepper and salt*
1 *teaspoon Worcestershire sauce*

1. Preheat oven to 400°F. Prick eggplant with sharp-pronged fork. Place on baking sheet and bake for 45 minutes. Let cool. Peel and dice.
2. Drop tomatoes into boiling water for 1 minute. Core and peel. Let cool. Dice.
3. In bowl, combine diced eggplant and tomato. Add balance of ingredients, one at a time, stirring gently after each addition (do not mash). For fully ripened flavor, store overnight in tightly sealed container.

YIELD: 2 cups; serving size = up to ½ cup

SERVING SUGGESTIONS: As an hors d'oeuvre, spread on thin whole-grain crackers; as a first course, serve on a bed of crisp lettuce leaves; as a relish, serve along with main course.

(95) CHOC-O-CHIP ICE MILK

½ cup skim milk
1¼ cups evaporated skim milk
½ cup unsweetened carob chips
2 tablespoons grain coffee

1 1-inch piece vanilla bean, split
¼ teaspoon ground cinnamon
3 tablespoons honey

1. Bring some water in bottom of double boiler to boil. Reduce heat to simmering. In top of double boiler, combine and stir skim milk, ¼ cup evaporated skim milk, ⅓ cup carob chips, grain coffee, vanilla bean, and cinnamon. Cook until chips are almost melted, about 4 minutes. Remove from heat. Stir in remaining chips. Let cool, stirring occasionally. Press out juices from vanilla bean, and discard bean.
2. Add honey and blend. Then stir in remaining 1 cup evaporated milk.
3. Pour into ice-cream maker, following manufacturer's directions, or pour into empty ice-cube trays. Turn refrigerator up to its coldest setting. Cover tray, and freeze, stirring from time to time. After 1 hour, briskly whisk or beat with portable electric beater or rotary mixer. Return to freezer until ice cream sets to desired consistency.

YIELD: About 1 pint; serving size = ½ cup

VARIATION: Pour mixture into Popsicle molds and freeze. Recipe will yield about 16 Popsicles.

Recipes Your Kids Can Make (Under Your Supervision)

There's no better way to get kids interested in eating bright, I believe, than by getting them interested in cooking my way. It's not hard. Cooking comes naturally to boys and girls. They don't regard it as a chore. It's fun, an exciting game with endless variations, surprises, and new delights. All the children in our family cook, and I think they're brighter for it, not only from the food, but from the mental stimulation that goes along with cooking. You know of course—and this is so important in getting kids to eat bright—kids love to eat what they make.

The recipes are listed here under Healthful "Junk-Food" Clones and New "Bright Cuisine" Recipes. References in **parentheses** are to recipe numbers. Actual recipes begin on page 183, and are arranged numerically. Those your kids can make (under your supervision) are distinguished there by a **K** preceding the title.

Healthful "Junk-Food" Clones

Tasty Muffins and Variations (3)
Pancakes and Variations (6)
Popcorn (9)
Whamburger (10)
Pizza Sauce (12)
French Fries (16)
Bread and Butter Pickles (18)
Ketchup De-Lite (19)
Salad Dressing (22)
Cheese Butter (23)
Applesauce (25)
Oatmeal Cookies (27)
Crunchy Candy Balls (28)
3-Juice Jell-O or Popsicles (29)

Creamy Mashed Potatoes (34A)
Colorful Mixed Vegetables (34A)
Brown Rice with Mushrooms (34B)
Steamed Peas (34B)
Pinto Beans (34C)
Crunchy Broccoli (34C)
"Fried" Chicken (36)
Lasagna (39)
Rice Mix (40)
Top-of-the-Stove Stuffing (41)
"Pouch-Type" Broccoli in Orange Sauce (42)
Barbecue Sauce (43)
Ice Cream Milk Shake (52)

New "Bright Cuisine" Recipes

Whole-Wheat Popovers (55)
Bacon-Tasting Onions and Eggs (56)
Stuffed Prunes (60)
Frozen Yogurt Tutti-Fruiti (61)
Veal Burger (64)

Versatile Sardine Salad (67)
Broccoli-Chicken Salad (71)
Colorful Salad with Fruit Dressing (72)
Peanut Butter Milk Shake (74)
Apple Sauté (76)

Cooking Terms Used in This Book

Al dente. Firm-textured. Said of pasta.

Bake. To cook in an oven with dry heat.

Barbecue. To cook on a grill or over hot coals or mesquite; or to combine ingredients to spread over food (marinate) to give it the taste of aforementioned cooking methods.

Baste. To spoon liquid over food while roasting or braising.

Batter. A liquid mixture comprised of such dry ingredients as flour and baking powder, and such liquids as eggs, milk, fruit juice, and so forth. Uncooked dough.

Blend. To combine two or more ingredients until well incorporated into each other.

Braise. To cook with a small amount of liquid over low heat, generally after food has been browned.

Broil. To cook uncovered under or over direct heat as in a broiler.

Brush. To cover a surface of food lightly with liquid, usually using a pastry brush.

Butterfly. Cut completely through backbone and spread apart.

Chill. To refrigerate food.

Chop. To cut into ⅛-inch cubes.

Coat. To cover a surface of food with another ingredient.

Combine. To stir together ingredients until evenly distributed.

Dash. Very small amount; about ¹⁄₁₆ teaspoon.

Dice. To cut into size-defined cubes; the cubes themselves.

Dot. Drop bits of butter over food.

Dredge. To coat food lightly with dry ingredients, generally shaking off excess.

Drizzle. To pour liquid in very fine stream all over surface of food.

Fillet. A boneless piece of meat, fish, or poultry.

Flake. Refers to the flesh of cooked fish that comes loose in flakes when touched with the tines of a fork. (Test for doneness.)

Florets. A small flower, one of a cluster without stem, such as in broccoli, cauliflower, parsley.

Fold in. A gentle method of combining a light mixture (such as whipped egg whites or cream) into a heavier mixture (such as cake batter).

Garnish. To decorate food with tasteful artistry.

Grate. Extremely small pieces of food obtained by rubbing on a grater.

Grease. To rub oil or other shortening on a pan, plate, or piece of waxed paper to prevent food from sticking.

Julienne. To cut food into matchstick pieces.

Knead. To press dough with hands in quarter-turn fold sequences until smooth and elastic.

Marinade. A seasoned liquid generally made up of vinegar, fruit juices, oil, herbs, and spices in which food soaks to tenderize and enhance flavors.

Mash. To crush to a soft mixture, as in mashed potatoes.

Mince. Cut into pieces smaller than ⅛-inch.

Poach. To gently cook in barely simmering broth.

Preheat. To turn oven on at a specified temperature 10 to 15 minutes before using.

Puree. To put food through a food mill, blender, or food processor to obtain a smooth-pulpy consistency.

Reduce. To continue cooking, usually over high heat in a pan, to concentrate liquid and, consequently, heighten flavor.

Roast. To cook poultry or meat by dry heat.

Sauté. To cook in a pan in a small amount of hot oil over low or medium heat.

Sift. To put through fine-meshed sieve or flour sifter.

Simmer. To cook just below boiling point over low heat.

Skim. To clear floating substances such as scum and fat from liquid.

Steam. To cook on a rack with steam rather than with liquid.

Stew. To slowly cook in simmering liquid in a covered pot.

Stir. Using a spoon, to combine food in a circular motion.

Tent. To cover food without pressure, using foil.

Toss. To mix with two utensils, as for salads.

Truss. To fasten the body of a fowl before cooking so that it holds its shape and cooks evenly.

Whisk. To beat rapidly in a circular motion using a wire whisk.

Utensils You Need

You probably have most of them in your cupboard now:

8- and 10-inch nonstick skillets with covers
8- to 10-inch iron skillet with cover (see instructions following this list for
    maintaining a well-seasoned iron skillet)
2-quart heavy-bottomed saucepan with cover
Food processor, large enough to hold up to 5 cups flour
Electric blender
Electric mixing machine
Vegetable steamer (inexpensive adjustable variety is fine)
Metal and rubber spatulas
Strainer
Medium-sized whisk
Double boiler
Sharp utility knife and sharpening steel
Paring knife
Serrated knife for cutting bread
10" x 15" jelly-roll pan
Muffin pan with 12 cups
Wire rack
Two 8-inch layer pans with removable bottoms
Four-sided grater
Ovenproof covered casserole
Shallow roasting pan
Food mill
Cutting board
Loaf pans
Swivel-bladed vegetable peeler
Slotted spoon
Nutmeg grater
Cotton cheesecloth
Pepper grinder

Instructions for well-seasoned iron skillet:

To keep your iron skillet well seasoned (which avoids sticking), wash in soapy water (do not soak). Dry thoroughly. Rub sparingly with oil. Place skillet over medium heat for 3 minutes, then let cool. Wipe out with paper toweling. Your skillet is now ready to use. After each use, wash in soapy water (do not use steel wool). Repeat seasoning process whenever skillet looks dry.

UTENSILS THAT WILL MAKE YOU AN EVEN BETTER COOK

Electric mayonnaise maker and herb chopper
Ice-cream making machine
Chinois (a conical-shaped fine-meshed metal sieve). It's a superb professional accessory for straining broths, stocks, ice cream, and sauces.

NOTE: All listed utensils are available in hardware or department stores.

Glossary

All technical terms are defined when first mentioned in the text (see Index). This is a glossary of key terms to be used as a rapid refresher.

AMINO ACIDS. Chemical building blocks of neurotransmitters. They're derived from proteins, and build proteins in the body/brain.

ANTI-MINERALS. Ingredients in foods, or the foods themselves, that inhibit the action of certain minerals in the body/brain.

ANTI-OXIDANTS. Certain vitamins, minerals, and amino acids that destroy oxidants, destructive biochemicals possibly activated in the body/brain by vitamin/mineral deficiencies.

ANTI-VITAMINS. Ingredients that act against vitamins as anti-minerals act against minerals.

CEREBRAL ALLERGENS. Substances in foods, or the foods themselves, that could cause brain disorders in children.

CHOLESTEROL. A brain-vital nutrient, especially for the child through age 5, it is also associated when in excess, or when improperly metabolized, with heart attacks and other degenerative diseases.

DENDRITES. Treelike structures at the tip of a nerve cell (neuron) that receive neurotransmitters.

DNA. A double-helix structure in each cell, holding the "blueprint" of the cell. The DNA in the nerve cells of the brain determine the basic construction of your child's brain, which can be altered by nutrition and stimulation.

FOOD GROUPS. Food arranged in groups in such a way that you can plan maximum-nutrition menus by making the right selections from each group.

FREE RADICALS. Destructive chemicals, probably produced by vitamin/mineral deficiencies in the body/brain leading to faulty metabolism. They scavenge all parts of the body, particularly the brain.

GLIAL-CELL COMPLEX. Glial cells and associated fatty structures responsible for feeding brain cells and protecting their electrical circuitry. They may be directly associated with intelligence.

GOITROGENS. Substances, mainly in food, which induce goiter, or preclinical symptoms of goiter, a disease associated with apathy, depression, and mental retardation.

JUNK FOOD. Food containing insufficient nutrients per calorie and/or harmful ingredients. Almost all processed foods are junk foods.

266

MINERALS. Inorganic materials, like iron and copper, necessary in small amounts for the functioning of the body/brain.

NEURON. The brain cell. The essential components are the nucleus, the dendrites, the axon, the "gates," the axon terminals, and the neurotransmitters. The nucleus contains the DNA. The dendrites receive neurotransmitter signals. The "gates" control the electric current that "fires" neurotransmitters from the cell. The axon terminals contain the neurotransmitters.

NEUROTRANSMITTER. A brain biochemical composed of amino acids, which carries signals activating or inhibiting sections of the brain responsible for specific activities. The former action is said to be "stimulatory," the latter "inhibitory." Some neurotransmitters are "stimulators," others are "inhibitors."

ODAs. Optimal Dietary Allowances of nutrients sufficient to prevent preclinical symptoms of a nutrient-deficiency disease.

OXIDANTS. See **FREE RADICALS.**

POLYUNSATURATED FATS. A group of fats containing the essential fatty acids, linoleic, linolenic, and arachidonic, necessary for the growth and maintenance of the glial-cell complex in your child's brain.

PRECLINICAL SYMPTOMS. Preliminary warning symptoms—such as fatigue, irritation, and general malaise—of a nutrient-deficiency disease. These preclinical symptoms are epidemic among Americans of all ages.

PROCESSED FRESH FOOD. Fresh food that's been treated with potentially harmful chemicals, biological agents, or procedures during growth, shipping, and storing.

RDAs. Recommended Dietary Allowances of nutrients sufficient to ward off clinical symptoms of nutrient-deficiency diseases but not preclinical symptoms.

SALICYLATES. Aspirinlike substances in foods that are associated with hyperactivity.

SATURATED FATS. A class of fats, mainly from animal sources, whose main function is to supply energy. They have been indicted as causative agents of heart attack and other degenerative diseases.

VITAMINS. Biochemicals vital in small quantities for vital processes of the body/brain.

Recommended Reading

These books have been selected for their readability and excellence. They are some of the sources for this book. There are thousands of scientific papers in the field of the nutrition/brain connection, far too many to be listed here. For references to any of these papers covering a specific subject, write to the authors in care of the publisher.

Allergies and the Hyperactive Child by Doris J. Rapp. New York: Cornerstone/ Simon & Schuster, 1981.

Allergy, Brains and Children Coping by Ray C. Wunderlich. St. Petersburg, Fla.: Johnny-Reads, 1973.

Amazing Amino Acids by William H. Lee. New Canaan, Conn.: Pivot/Keats, 1984.

The Amazing Brain by Robert Ornstein and Richard F. Thompson. Boston: Houghton Mifflin, 1984.

Amino Acids Book by Carlson Wade. New Canaan, Conn.: Pivot/Keats, 1985.

Are You Allergic? by William G. Crook. Jackson, Tenn.: Professional Books, 1978.

The Baby Checkup Book by Sheilah Hillman. New York: Bantam, 1982.

The Biology of Human Fetal Growth, D. F. Roberts and A. M. Thomson, editors. New York: Halstead, 1976.

Body, Mind, and the B Vitamins by Ruth Adams and Frank Murray. New York: Larchmont, 1979.

The Book of Vitamin Therapy by Harold Rosenberg and A. N. Feldzaman. New York: Berkley Books, 1975.

The Brain by Richard Restak. New York: Bantam, 1984.

The Brain Food Diet for Children by Ralph E. Minear. New York: Bobbs-Merrill, 1983.

Breastfeeding: A Manual for Health Professionals by V. A. LaCerva. New York: Medical Examination Publications, 1981.

The Broken Brain by Nancy C. Andreason. New York: Harper & Row, 1984.

The Brown Bag Cookbook by Sara Sloan. Charlotte, Vt.: Williamson, 1984.

Can Your Child Read? Is He Hyperactive? by William G. Crook. Jackson, Tenn.: Professional Books, 1978.

Child Development and Personality by Paul H. Mussen, John J. Conger, and Jerome Kagan. New York: Harper & Row, 1969.

Children Cook Naturally by Sara Sloan. Atlanta, Ga.: Nutra Program, 1980.

Child's Body by The Diagram Group. New York: Wallaby/Simon & Schuster, 1977.

Choline, Lecithin, Inositol and Other "Accessory" Nutrients by Jeffrey Bland. New Canaan, Conn.: Keats, 1982.

From Classroom to Cafeteria: A Nutrition Guide for Teachers and Managers by Sara Sloan. Atlanta, Ga.: Nutra Program, 1978.

The Complete Guide to Anti-Aging Nutrients by Sheldon Saul Hendler. New York: Simon & Schuster, 1985.

The Conscious Brain by Steven Ross. New York: Knopf, 1973.

Creative Food Experiences with Children by Mary T. Goodwin and Gerry Pollan. Washington, D.C.: Center for Science in the Public Interest, 1980.

Day-by-Day Baby Care by Miriam Stoppard. New York: Villard/Random House, 1983.

The Development of the Brain by S. Reines and J. M. Goldman. Springfield, Ill.: Thomas, 1980.

Deviant Children Grow Up by L. Robins. Baltimore, Md.: Williams and Wilkins, 1966.

Diet and Disease by E. Cheraskin, W. M. Ringsdorf, and J. W. Clark. New Canaan, Conn.: Keats, 1968.

Diet, Crime and Delinquency by Alexander G. Schauss. Berkeley, Ca.: Parker House, 1980.

A Diet for Living by Jean Mayer. New York: David McKay, 1975.

Dr. Cott's Help for Your Learning Disabled Child by Alan Cott. New York: Times Books, 1985.

Dr. Spock's Baby and Child Care by Benjamin Spock and Michael B. Rothanberg. New York: Bantam, 1985.

Feed Your Kids Right by Lendon Smith. New York: Dell, 1979.

The Food Depression Connection by June Roth. Chicago: Contemporary, 1978.

Foods for Healthy Kids by Lendon Smith. New York: McGraw-Hill, 1981.

Growth and Development of the Brain: Nutrition, Genetics, Environment, M. A. B. Brazier, editor. New York: Raven Press, 1975.

A Guide for Nutra Lunches and Natural Foods by Sara Sloan. Atlanta, Ga.: Nutra Program, 1977.

The Healing Factor by Irwin Stone. New York: Grosset & Dunlap, 1974.

Healthy Living in an Unhealthy World by Edward J. Calabrese and Michael W. Dorsey. New York: Simon & Schuster, 1984.

How to Improve Your Child's Behavior Through Diet by Laura J. Stevens and Rosemary B. Stoner. New York: Doubleday, 1979.

How to Live with Schizophrenia by Abram Hoffer and Humphrey Osmond. Secaucus, N.J.: University Books, 1974.

Improving Your Child's Behavior Chemistry by Lendon Smith. Englewood Cliffs, N.J.: Prentice-Hall, 1976.

Infant and Child Feeding, J. T. Bond, editor. New York: Academic Press, 1981.

Infant Nutrition, D. H. Merritt, editor. New York: Halstead/Wiley, 1978.

Infants and Mothers by T. Berry Brazelton. New York: Delacorte/Lawrence, 1983.

Lysine, Tryptophan and Other Amino Acids by Robert Garrison, Jr. New Canaan, Conn.: Keats, 1982.

Mega-Nutrients for Your Nerves by H. L. Newbold. New York: Wydon, 1975.

Mega-Vitamin Therapy by Ruth Adams and Frank Murphy. New York: Larchmont, 1973.

Mental and Elemental Nutrients by Carl Pfeiffer. New Canaan, Conn.: Keats, 1977.

Mind, Mood and Medicine by Paul H. Wender and Donald F. Klein. New York: Farrar, Strauss, Giroux, 1981.

Neuronal Man by Jeanne-Pierre Changeux. New York: Pantheon/Random House, 1985.

Nursing Your Baby by Karen Pryor. New York: Harper & Row, 1963.

Nutrition by Cheryl Corbin. New York: Holt, Rinehart & Winston, 1981.

Nutrition Against Disease by Roger S. Williams. New York: Bantam, 1981.

Nutritional Parenting by Sara Sloan. New Canaan, Conn.: Keats, 1982.

Nutrition Almanac by John D. Kirschmann and Lavon S. Dunne. New York: McGraw-Hill, 1984.

Nutritional Impacts on Women Throughout Life with Emphasis on Reproduction by K. S. Moghissi and T. N. Evans. Hagerstrum, Md.: Harper & Row, 1977.

Nutrition and Child Health Perspectives for the 1980's, R. C. Tsang and B. L. Nichols, Jr., editors. New York: Alan R. Liss, 1980.

Nutrition and Growth, D. Jelliffe and E. F. P. Jelliffe, editors. New York: Plenum, 1979.

Nutrition and Mental Function, G. Serban, editor. New York: Plenum, 1975.

Nutrition and Physical Degeneration by Weston Price. Santa Monica, Ca.: Price-Pottinger Foundation, 1970.

Nutrition and Your Child's Behavior by Hugh Powers and James Pressley. New York: St. Martin's Press, 1978.

Nutrition and Your Mind by George Watson. New York: Harper & Row, 1974.

The Nutrition Business by John Yudkin. New York: St. Martin's Press, 1968.

Nutrition, Development and Social Behavior. Washington, D. C.: U.S. Government Printing Office, DHEW, [NIH], 1973.

Nutrition in Infancy and Childhood by P. Piper. St. Louis, Mo.: Mosby, 1977.

Nutrition in the 1980's, N. Selvey and P. L. White, editors. New York: Alan R. Liss, 1981.

The Orthomolecular Approach to Learning Disabilities by Alan Cott. San Rafael, Ca.: Academic Therapy, 1977.

Orthomolecular Nutrition: New Lifestyle for Super Good Health by Abram Hoffer. New Canaan, Conn.: Pivot/Keats, 1978.

Overcoming Learning Disabilities by Martin Baren, Robert Liebl, and Lendon Smith. Reston, Va.: Reston, 1978.

Parent's Guide to Nutrition by Boston Children's Hospital. Boston: Addison Wesley, 1986.

The Pediatric Guide to Drugs and Vitamins by Edward R. Brace. New York: Delacorte/Stonesong, 1982.

Pediatrics, H. L. Barnett, editor. New York: Appleton-Century-Croft/Prentice Hall, 1972.

A Physician's Handbook on Orthomolecular Medicine, R. J. Williams and D. K. Kalita, editors. New York: Pergamon, 1977.

Pregnancy and Nutrition by Miriam Erick. Brookline, Mass.: Grinnen-Barrett, 1984.

Present Knowledge of Nutrition, 5th edition, by Robert E. Olson, Chairman, Editorial Committee. Washington, D.C.: The Nutrition Foundation, 1984.

The Psychobiology of Aggression by K. E. Mayer. New York: Harper & Row, 1976.

Psychodietetics by E. Cheraskin and W. M. Ringsdorf. New York: Bantam, 1976.

Psycho-Nutrition by Carlton Fredericks. New York: Grosset & Dunlap, 1976.

RNA and Brain Function, Memory and Learning, M. A. B. Brazier, editor. Berkeley, Los Angeles: University of California Press, 1964.

The Saccharine Disease by T. L. Cleave. New Canaan, Conn.: Keats, 1975.

Something's Wrong with My Child by Milton Brutten, Sylvia O. Richardson, and Charles Mangel. New York: Harcourt Brace Jovanovich, 1973.

Sugar Blues by William Duffy. New York: Warner Books, 1975.

Supernutrition by Richard J. Passwater. New York: Dial, 1975.

A Textbook of Pediatric Nutrition, D. S. McLaren and D. Burman, editors. New York: Churchill/Livingston, 1982.

The Total Nutrition Guide for Mother and Baby by Alice White. New York: Ballantine/Random House, 1983.

Trace Minerals by Erwin DiCyan. New Canaan, Conn.: Keats, 1984.

The Universe Within by Morton Hunt. New York: Simon & Schuster, 1982.

Vitamin Bible for Your Kids by Earl Mindell. New York: Bantam, 1982.

The Vitamin Book by Rick Wentzler. New York: Dolphin/Doubleday, 1979.

The Vitamin Robbers by Earl Mindell and William H. Lee. New Canaan, Conn.: Keats, 1983.

Vitamins and You by Robert J. Benowicz. New York: Berkley Books, 1981.

Why Your Child Is Hyperactive by Ben F. Feingold. New York: Random House, 1974.

Woman's Body by The Diagram Group. New York: Wallaby/Simon & Schuster, 1977.

Your Child and Vitamin E by Wilfrid E. Shute. New Canaan, Conn.: Pivot/ Keats, 1979.

Your Child's Sensory World by Lise Liepmann. New York: Dial, 1973.

Your Personal Vitamin Profile by Michael Colgan. New York: Quill/Morrow, 1982.

Zinc and Other Micro-Nutrients by Carl C. Pfeiffer. New Canaan, Conn.: Keats, 1978.

Index

About the Authors

Francine Prince is the author of the book that started the nutrition revolution in the kitchen. Her internationally acclaimed best-selling *Dieter's Gourmet Cookbook* introduced her "gourmet cuisine of health"—the first, and still the only, cuisine truly low in fat/saturated fat, high in fiber, without a grain of sugar or salt, and as stingy in calories as it's extravagant in taste. With six extremely successful subsequent books on cooking for better health, numerous articles in national publications, more than 1,000 appearances on TV and radio, and a large devoted following, Francine Prince has become the leading exponent of cooking right—and now, cooking bright.

Harold Prince, a Ph.D. in biochemistry, is most recently the behind-the-scenes author of the best-selling *I Love New York Diet* with Bess Myerson and *The I Love America Diet* with Phyllis George. He is a prolific writer in the fields of nutrition, medicine, and science, and several of his works under other bylines have been major book club selections, excerpted in national magazines, and translated into foreign languages. A protagonist of better health through better food, he has written innovative books on the dietary approach to heart attack, skin care, general health and fitness; and on nutritional therapy as opposed to drug therapy for women and children.

The Princes, a husband-and-wife team, are native New Yorkers.